MCO
LA...2021

Walking With Anthony

A MOTHER'S FIGHT FOR HER SON

MICKI PURCELL

WALKING WITH ANTHONY: A MOTHER'S FIGHT FOR HER SON

Published by TVGuestpert Publishing

ISBN-13: ISBN - 978-1-7358981-0-0

BISAC CODES: BIO033000, HEA018000, HEA028000

Nationwide Distribution through Ingram & New Leaf Distributing Company.

This publication is designed to provide accurate and authoritative information in regards to the subject matter covered. It is sold with the understanding that the publisher is not engaged in rendering legal, accounting, or other professional service. If legal advice or other expert assistance is required, the services of a competent professional person should be sought. – From a Declaration of Principles

Jointly adopted by a committee of the American Bar Association and a committee of Publishers and Associations.

Some names and identifying details have been changed to protect the privacy of individuals. All brand names, product names, and team names used in this book are trademarks, registered trademarks or trade names of their respective holders.

TVGuestpert Publishing and the TVG logo are trademarks of Jacquie Jordan Inc.

TVGuestpert & TVGuestpert Publishing are subsidiaries of Jacquie Jordan Inc.

TVGuestpert & TVGuestpert Publishing are visionary media companies that seek to educate, enlighten, and entertain the masses with the highest level of integrity. Our full-service production company, publishing house, management, and media development firm promises to engage you creatively and honor you and ourselves, as well as the community, in order to bring about fulfillment and abundance both personally and professionally.

Front Book Cover Design by Jonathan Fong
Book Design by Carole Allen Design Studio
Author Photos by Kate Haus Photography
Edited by TVGuestpert Publishing
Published by TVGuestpert Publishing

11664 National Blvd, #345
Los Angeles, CA 90064
310-584-1504
www.TVGuestpertPublishing.com
www.TVGuestpert.com

First Printing November 2020

10 9 8 7 6 5 4 3 2 1

Walking with Anthony

A MOTHER'S FIGHT FOR HER SON

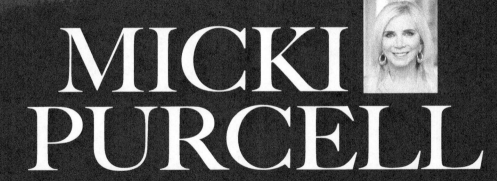

MICKI
PURCELL

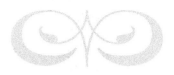

Psalm 55:22

"Cast your burden on the Lord, and he will sustain you, he will never permit the righteous to be moved."

To my son Anthony ~

Nothing could have prepared me for the journey we have shared together, and I couldn't be more proud of the man that you have become.

I wrote this book in honor of your unwavering courage, determination, and perseverance—and your continuous fight for the higher advocacy of all who struggle in the spinal cord injury (SCI) community.

You are a true inspiration to me and those who have been touched by you.

I am honored to be your Mother, your advocate, and your Walking With Anthony partner.

I love you with all my heart.

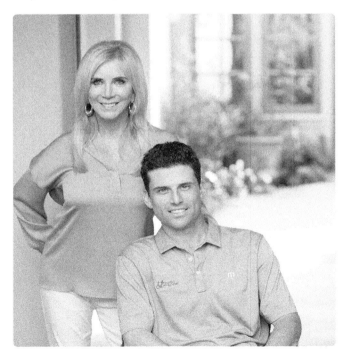

To my family –

My daughter, Jennifer, and my son-in-law, Matt. My grandchildren Makayla, Mackenzie, and Matthew. You are my heart.

My absolute angel, Karen…of course, Anthony's too.

Joe, thank you for being a great father to our children and never leaving Anthony's side.

Michael & Rita, Joseph & Sloan, thank you for your love and support.

My Nolan siblings — Pat & Loretta, Terry & Barry, Joanne & Bryan, Frannie & Bernie, Bernie and Debbie, Chrissy, Tommy, Barbara & Ted, Billy, Katy and their families for all their continual support and love.

My mother, also known as Gigi, thank you for showing me the example of how to be a strong woman; and to my father, whose spirit has never left my heart through all of this.

My niece Tonya Kowalcyck, thank you from the bottom of my heart for your steadfast commitment to Walking With Anthony and your continued love and dedication for this cause.

My nephew Bernie McKeever, I couldn't have written this book if you hadn't saved Anthony's life.

My nephew Tommy Nolan, my Godson, who put his life on hold and has been by Anthony's side the entire journey with endless love and support.

My nephew Kyle McKeever, whose heart of unconditional love was the best gift you could give Anthony.

My sister Frannie & brother-in-law Bernie McKeever, who have always been there for me and have always given their hearts and souls to Walking With Anthony.

My nieces and nephews: Re & Geoff, Matt & Erin, Tonya, Deanna, Melissa, Bernie & Heather, Kyle, Kellie, Bernie & Katrina, Alexandra, Tom, Patrick & Linda, Colleen & Grant, Erin & Ralph, Tommy & Katie, Micki, Natalie, Teddy, Caroline, Sydney, Billy Jr., Shannon & Troy, Theresa & Will, Sean & Carrie, and Heather & Bridget – for all your prayers and support.

And a special thanks to Anthony's cousins, Joey Haynos and Tommy McCarthy, for all your love and support.

To our support and wellness team –

Dr. Allan Levi, Chairman of Neurosurgery at the University of Miami MILLER School of Medicine, who performed the life-saving emergency surgery on Anthony the day of his accident.

Dr. Barth Green, Co-Founder and Chairman of the Miami Project to

Cure Paralysis, for his innovative expertise of spinal cord injury.

Lulu & Cheryl, Anthony's nurses who are still friends with us today and who were instrumental in getting both Anthony's body and soul fed on a daily basis with care and compassion during his hospital stay.

Marie & Mike, who were Anthony's occupational and physical therapists and who rooted him on during his rehab at Jackson Memorial Hospital.

Norma Macias, who aids Anthony every day to ensure he lives his best possible life.

Ted Dardzinski, founder of Project Walk, who gave Anthony the foundation and knowledge to learn the fundamentals of a strong recovery.

Mike Barwis, founder and CEO of Barwis Methods, who inspired, motivated, and taught Anthony the method of physical rehab that Anthony uses every day.

Janne Kouri, founder of NextStep, who participated in Anthony's recovery and has become one of Walking With Anthony's national resources to help other spinal cord injury victims get the rehabilitation they need.

To the Washington Redskins organization, currently known as Washington Football Team -

Dan & Tanya Snyder, Washington Redskins owner,

Bruce Allen, former team president of the Washington Redskins,

Jerry Olsen, executive director of the Redskins Alumni Association,

Rick "Doc" Walker, former NFL player turned radio sports commentator,

Larry Michael, the former voice of the Washington Redskins,

Jane Rodgers, former executive director of the Washington Redskins Charitable Foundation,

Terri Lamb, the president of the Washington Redskins Cheerleaders Alumni Association, for bringing in the First Ladies of Football Cheerleaders,

A special thanks to Vernon Davis, former Washington Redskins tight end, LaVar Arrington, former Washington Redskins linebacker, and all the Washington Redskins alumni who have consistently participated,

Thanks for joining hands with us for this very important cause. Your support has been invaluable.

To our athletic event participators -

Tommy Fitzgerald, Walking With Anthony's Annual Golf Tournament Event Director,

Chris Blanchard, president of MTM Group,

Jerry West, former NBA great of the LA Lakers and current NBA Executive,

Tom Thibodeau, former Chicago Bulls' head coach,

Anthony Fasano, former Miami Dolphins tight end,

John Buck, former Florida Marlins catcher,

Neal Wilkinson, former Green Bay Packers tight end and founder of Open-Field Foundation,

John Salley, former professional NBA player and talk show host,

Kevin Everett, former Buffalo Bills tight end,

Gabby Sanchez, former Pittsburgh Pirates first baseman,

Without whom we couldn't have come this far without your participation.

To Anthony's many endearments -

Anthony's friends who have always been there for him, even in the most difficult of times, including Bill Doody, Sean Swartz, Derek Stoller, Joey Fitzgerald, Ben Greaves, Marcus Cortese (Boomer), Chris Holker, and Dexter Lewis.

Special Thanks -

My friends Karen West and Lori Cortese for your unwavering love and support during this challenging journey,

Richard Waner for encouraging me for years to write this book and share this journey of Walking With Anthony.

To our Walking With Anthony heroes -

All the heroes — WWA Warriors, who have survived and thrived with Spinal Cord Injury, know that we are with you throughout your journey. .

To my almighty God –

Thank you for giving me the strength, spiritual guidance and emotional courage to carry me through this blessed transformation.

Table of Contents

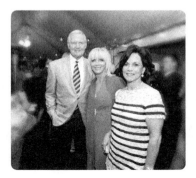

When we first met Micki Purcell almost forty years ago, we knew she was unique, like a whirlwind just entered your space. Her personality is BIG, as is her drive and determination. Everyone knows when Micki is in proximity—there is nothing demure about her. You either love her or you hate her but you will never forget her. She voices her opinion loud and clear and will not take no for an answer. Our personalities are completely opposite yet we became fast friends. A friendship that has never wavered.

Luckily for Anthony Purcell she is his mother because when Anthony suffered a spinal cord injury while diving into the ocean, Micki went into high gear and there was never a time that anyone dared to say no to her demands. With Micki as his advocate, Anthony received the best care while in the hospital. While on his road to recovery, she pushed and pleaded and pushed some more—to a point that some people would run when they saw her coming.

Everyone should be lucky enough to have someone like Micki on their side when in a troubling situation. With Micki to fight for Anthony, he has made strides that the medical community didn't think possible. Anthony takes after his mother as he is strong and has worked diligently to be the best man that he can be. His continuous hard work has paid off and thankfully his darkest days are behind him. Anthony is a loving husband to his wife Karen, an unwavering advocate for the SCI community, a successful businessman, and the life of the party—just like his mom.

As you read their story, you will see Anthony's and Micki's passion and compassion to fight for better health care and rights for people with disabilities, and in particular for those who have suffered spinal cord injuries. It's a long battle but if anyone can get it accomplished we'd bet on Micki.

Karen West, Walking With Anthony Board Member
Jerry West, Legendary NBA Hall of Famer and Executive

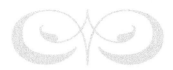

Psalm 56:3

"When I am afraid, I put my trust in thee."

Introduction

You probably don't know me. We may not have a lot in common. However, if you are reading this book, we most likely share one very big thing in common. I am a parent. Like all mothers and fathers, I will do anything to help my child. And I am a mother who has had to help my adult child through a very difficult time. No matter how old your child is, he or she is always your child.

The story that I am about to share with you in *Walking With Anthony* may not be the same as yours. But I'm positive you have had to fight for the well-being of your child at one time or another, and I'm betting that at times you felt very alone. Hopefully, your child has not been through the same, or similar, life trauma as Anthony or the other Heroes we meet later in this book, but trust me when I say, from parent to parent, you and I have much in common in our battles.

I have been fighting for my adult son's well-being for the last seven years endlessly, and our fight continues. I wouldn't wish my journey on anyone. Writing this book is only one way I am speaking out about the many battles parents, people with disabilities, and spinal cord victims face on a daily basis. I will not stop until something is done to make some real positive change. I am not Anthony's voice; however, I am Anthony's advocate.

For that matter, I'm working to get in front of our own United States President. I have been able to prove over and over again that people just like my son can benefit from the kind of help I gave him. They get healthier, grow stronger, and get their independence back. Many of them have had the medical society turn their backs on them. Being ignored does not help the individual, their family or the nation as a whole. I would show the President the video of our compelling success stories and the results we get from our work.

No one wants to give up on someone in a wheelchair, whether it's a child or an adult. I bet you're rolling your eyes as you read this thinking my dream is too big, but I'll say exactly what I said when people told me I couldn't possibly start a charity with my son Anthony at the helm:

"Just. You. Watch!"

If I could have just ten minutes in front of the President, it would change the lives of spinal cord victims forever. Until then, enjoy my book.

Micki Purcell

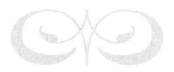

Psalm 118:6

"With the Lord on my side, I do not fear."

CHAPTER ONE

Sudden Impact

I was driving over the speed limit. Just a little. Unusual for the 405 Interstate in Southern California. Unusual for me. I respect limits, but limits don't hold me back.

My sister Frannie and I were on our way to the Northern Trust Golf Tournament that Jerry West was hosting at the Riviera Golf Club in Brentwood, California. Jerry and his wife, Karen, have been dear friends of mine for forty years. From the passenger seat, I could see Frannie shuffle through her purse that sat on the floor of my car as we heard her cell phone ringing. Just by the ringtone, I knew it was my nephew Bernie. As we were getting close to our destination, northbound, to the Sunset Boulevard exit, Frannie started to scream.

"What? Speak slower. Anthony? How bad?" Frannie croaked out loud muffled screams, as she tried to make sense of what Bernie was telling her. While I continued to drive, I gathered from her that Anthony, my only son, was in an ambulance and that Bernie had just saved his life. I was unable to fully comprehend what happened and how my life was about to suddenly change. What did the pieces of everything I just heard even mean? The moment didn't hit me hard at first.

Sunset to the overpass and back to the 405, a U-turn, as I knew instinctively to head south to LAX, the Los Angeles International Airport. Frantically passing cell phones back and forth, Frannie and I booked the next flight to Miami. Panic began to ensue in me as we tried to catch an emergency flight.

I heard, "Press one for English," "Press three for flight reservations," and "Please stay on hold for an agent representative who will be on with you in a moment." Then I listened to the never-ending music.

I had actually been happy to be in Los Angeles and was looking forward to catching up with some of my old friends. Miami was hosting the Superbowl that same weekend, so it seemed everyone and their mother was in South Florida, our home. Booking a last-minute ticket was not going to be easy, or so I thought. Luck did come our way; there were literally two seats left. *Thank God*, a blessing in the middle of a blur.

As a mother, when your kid is happy, you're happy. Any mother can attest to that. The last conversation I had with Anthony was at 10am, Los Angeles time.

Anthony and I are close. We just are. He and I have that mother-son bond. I unconditionally love my daughter just

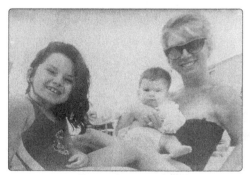

Jennifer, Anthony, and Micki

as much, of course. I love my grandbabies too, but Anthony and I just have this indescribable connection...we just do.

While driving to the airport and thinking of Anthony, I flashed back to when I was resolutely the first mother in line at the grade school carpool to pick up Anthony. I did this every single day without fail. I scheduled my entire workday to get that front spot for him. Naturally, it was at Anthony's request. "No matter what Mom!" he would demand.

My mind also floated back to Anthony playing high school basketball at St. Coleman's, my "Mr. Three-pointer" star. He wouldn't energetically warm-up at the game until I walked into the gymnasium. Once he spotted me, he would get jazzed up and ready to play. I was his biggest fan, his biggest supporter, and he knew it.

The night before this current life-changing accident, Anthony was living the best life. He had attended a huge ESPN party and was excited to watch the Saints play against the Colts at Hard Rock Stadium. Bernie, who is one of many of Anthony's cousins, played at The University of Virginia, and Anthony's other cousin, Joey Haynos, played for the Miami Dolphins, which gave Anthony plus-one access to a lucky night of spectacular Super Bowl parties. This even included a Maxim party that any guy in their early twenties would have traded their left foot for. The last thing Anthony said to me in our casual conversation that particular morning was that he had the best time of his life, ever. The Miami high life was what Anthony was fortunate to be living.

Bernie, a 200+ pound linebacker, and Anthony always swam together in the ocean. You could find them anywhere; whether it was Ocean City, Maryland (near where I grew up) or Fort Lauderdale. They even went up and down the Atlantic ocean. These boys weren't ones to miss the waves if they had the chance to dive in.

As fate made it that day, Bernie decided it was too cold to swim, which was unusual. Undeterred, Anthony did a body-surf dive into an inviting wave, wanting to experience the ocean on his skin and take in the salt water after a night he called, "The best night of my life." Looking back now, Anthony would be dead if Bernie hadn't stayed on the shore. Anthony also would have died, if Bernie weren't so strong or so big.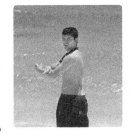

Then the glamour dissipated like a shooting star extinguishes. Bernie thought it was a joke when he saw Anthony floating in the water just ten feet from the shore. After all, it happened fast. Bernie had just turned away to walk back to the shore line to escape the cold water, and when he turned back around he just saw...

Anthony.

Face down.

Floating.

Then, with startling realization, *Oh, shit!*, he dove in.

Sudden impact. The moment that changed all our lives forever.

You hear about swimming accidents all the time. You may not hear about swimming accidents involving sandbars often, but they do happen and can have dire consequences. Sandbars are ripples of sand under the water like moving sand castles. People typically think of sandbars as beautiful sand islands that you might find somewhere like Fiji or Bora Bora, where you can see your feet in the water. People don't think of sandbars paralyzing someone. But the Atlantic water is darker than it is for most other surf bays. It's not like you can easily see your feet on an unpredictably migrating sand floor surface created by strong waves. Anthony's accident happened not even ten feet from the shore line. In rough waves, the sand floor can recreate itself into an unexpected gorge terrain, where you assume it's flat and slowly descending only to tragically find out, like Anthony did, it's a brick wall under the water.

Since the underwater terrain is always migrating, it's not easy for city officials to notify swimmers of its perils. Where Anthony was, there were no warning flags, signs, or lifeguards for swimmers to know of the moving sandbars. Often flags reflect rip tides and currents, but only sometimes sandbars.

Anthony's spinal cord injury didn't just affect Anthony. It affected our entire family. Shock waves of change reached further than just his internal family. Ripples ran through and were felt by our entire extended family. Waves of tears ran through all Anthony's twenty-eight cousins and my ten brothers and sisters. None of our lives have ever been the same. And, of course, it goes without mentioning, Anthony's life hasn't been the same, nor is Anthony even the same person.

As I slammed my brakes to park at the airport parking lot, I still didn't feel any emotion. Shuffling to get my belongings together and my head screwed on right, I felt outright clueless, which is not normal for me. Keys? Check. Golf shoes can stay in the car. Do I have my overnight? Do I care? What am I thinking? What am I feeling? What I did know was, this was going to be the longest flight of my life.

To calm my nerves, I ordered a vodka on the rocks in the stuffy cabin. I'm not usually the quietest person in the room, and at this moment, I was not paying attention to how loud I was actually speaking. As my sister and I rehashed the story that Bernie frantically told her over the phone, chewing every piece of it like a morsel that our mouths would rather choke on than swallow, a few people on our flight shared their unsolicited input. Specifically, the man seated behind us chimed in declaring that our description of Anthony's accident was a sign of being paralyzed. The movie star looking guy next to me displayed a tremendous amount of compassion. Chivalrously, he came to my defense, telling the guy behind us that his assumptions weren't necessarily true.

He reassuringly touched my arm, looked at me, and said, "Your son is going to be fine."

I chose to believe him. That's what I do. If there are two ways to look at things — the *good way* or the *bad way* — I will find a way to make it the *good way* and I hope to spread and share this positive light with others.

Sudden impact. As soon as the plane touched down, I was able to get cell phone service again. I called my daughter Jennifer, Anthony's only sister, who had already been at the hospital for several hours. Then it all hit me. It hit me hard. I went crashing down like a sack of potatoes.

"It's bad, mom, it's really bad," said Jennifer, who I could tell was really shook up. As a mom knows, when I heard my daughter's voice, I knew it was bad.

Before the door opened on the plane, I fainted at Jennifer's *bad way of sharing* Anthony's update. Jennifer, Anthony's older sister by seven years, was the first to arrive at the hospital. She was the one making all the moment-to-moment decisions with the guidance of their dad, Joe, while he boarded his own flight. Jennifer sent Anthony into emergency surgery without my presence or Joe's, while we scrambled to travel cross country. While I had my airplane fainting episode, Joe sobbed during his own flight from Southern California with my niece, Tonya, and nephew, Kyle, who sat behind him on the plane marinating in their own fears.

God bless her. We had just celebrated Jennifer's thirtieth birthday nine days earlier at the Riverside Hotel in Fort Lauderdale on February 1st. It was the last time I danced with my son before the accident; now it's a memory etched forever into my brain. Before I rushed off the plane, the last words I heard Jennifer say were, "The Doctor says it is the worst case he has ever seen. He may or may not make it."

After waking up on the dirty airplane floor, I was slowly guided by the handsome man sitting next to me on the airplane. I was brought back to reality by Brad Pitt. It was a surreal moment on top of another surreal moment. I wished he could have made my nightmare reality go away. I never had a chance to thank him, but he was a true gentleman for giving me comfort in a time of need. He was on our same flight because he was taking his own son, Maddox, to the Super Bowl.

I was simply blindsided by the events of the day, and I wanted to focus on staying in my body and focus on my son's well-being. I chose to hail a cab with Frannie. All the while, our family began to gather at Jackson Memorial.

I remember my panic when Anthony was just a baby. He projectile vomited on me and it scared me to death as a new mother, especially when Joe was out of town. I remember how catastrophic that moment was for me because he was a baby and needed to be cared for in every way possible. So, like what any panicky mother does when she thinks her baby is sick, I drove Anthony to the doctor for a checkup, which turned out fine.

Upon entering the hospital, I breathed deeply so as not to overwhelm myself with how catastrophic the moment was, because I didn't really know what I was walking into. The waiting room was packed with familiar faces: immediate family, loved ones, solid and stoic friends of mine, friends of Anthony from the previous night, from high school, from sports. Of course, all I could think about was getting past everyone and going directly to Anthony.

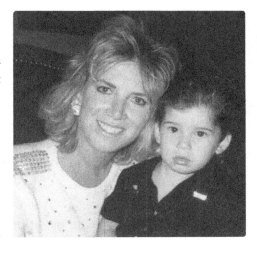

Coming from a large family, I am used to large living rooms, large celebrations, large receptions, large crowds, loud voices, and noisy rooms. Through the sea of it all, what stood out was my friend Lori's look of terror. Lori arrived soon after Jennifer and her husband, Matt, and Boomer, one of Anthony's closest friends. As everyone walked up to me with a mixed wave of confusion and comfort, I walked instead straight towards the elevator and let everything and everyone else fade into a blur as I made my way to my son's side.

"Anthony," I whispered.

Life or death. Every moment counted. Anthony had been taken immediately into surgery to fuse his C4 and C5 vertebrae, performed by Dr. Allan Levi. Luckily, Dr. Levi was in Miami for the Super Bowl. As luck would have it, he was on call should any NFL players be injured with similar injuries as Anthony.

Just like when I was first in line at school in the carpool pick-up lane, I was the first person by his side when he came out of surgery. I was devastated to see my son with a medical halo on his head and scared of what was to come next. Still, I thought, *Thank God*. No, I really mean, *Thank God*. Anthony survived the surgery.

This moment was tragic, but it was nothing when compared to what lay ahead of us.

I would stay with Anthony until he finally woke up, which wasn't for several days. Even while he slept, I kissed his cheeks, spoke reassurances to him, anything that let him know I was there with him even if he couldn't open his eyes. Minutes bled into hours and hours into days. Even with the relief of his surviving the accident and the surgery, I had no idea what trauma may lay ahead of us. Then one day, he finally opened his eyes.

"Hi, honey! You're going to be okay, Anthony," I went right into the reassurances while holding his hand. No room for doubt or fear, his or mine.

It was in that moment when I sobered up into my new role as mother/advocate.

Look at all the support Anthony and I had in the hospital with family and friends. Everyone needs an advocate in an emergency situation. The U.S. healthcare system is not set up to advocate for patients. If Anthony hadn't landed specifically at Jackson Memorial Hospital, he wouldn't have had the cutting edge spinal cord procedure, developed by Dr. Barth Green, and performed by the great Dr. Allan Levi. Dr. Green, whose focus is spinal cord injury, is from the Miami Project, and is a professor and chairman of the Department of Neurosurgery at the University of Miami. If you have this type of accident in Timbuktu, what do you do? Who do you turn to?

We had support. We had the resources, but this journey still was not easy. Our learning curve was steep. The consequences in decision making were immediate and severe. I had to dig deep and acclimate fast to ensure my son would not waste away. Every minute, every decision mattered, and I would not let my lack of knowledge be the reason for Anthony's chances of survival.

That's what a spine does...it supports. Theoretically, when you have no spine, you have no support. Who do you, and other families, lean on in emergencies? You can't count on the medical community.

You can't depend on the hospitals. It's definitely not going to be the insurance companies. The journey of a family member with a spinal cord injury is brutal, absolutely horrific, ruthless, and life destroying beyond anything you can even imagine. That's also what survival looks like, not just for the patient but for every loved one of the injured. It just doesn't have to be this way.

———◆———

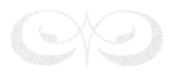

Joshua 1:9

"Have I not commanded you? Be strong and of good courage, be not frightened, neither be dismayed, for the Lord your God is with you wherever you go."

CHAPTER TWO

A Slow Burn

Reality started to seep in. The noise of the machines. The sights and sounds. The alarms constantly sounding on and off. Adrenalin starts to fade. Rinse and Repeat. A slowing down of my reality as the outside world no longer existed. The next thirty days were spent in the ICU with Anthony.

Jennifer, dizzy from emotional exhaustion, paced the halls mumbling about a family curse that she believed has been cast upon us.

I overheard her saying, "I knew our lives were too charmed, too easy, too perfect. Something bad had to happen."

We couldn't comprehend how an accident of this magnitude could happen to Anthony. He didn't deserve it. But accidents can happen to anyone.

Jennifer had been the first to arrive at the hospital and was burdened with the task, as I mentioned before, of making the life-threatening - turned lifesaving - decisions for Anthony before either Joe or I arrived on the scene. Jennifer was now in a state of emotional hangover, and rightfully so, as the sobering reality set in for all of us.

Drip. Drip. Drip. Drip. Drops of saline in the IV passed through the clear tubing into Anthony's arm in a clock-ticking manner. I heard screams from other ICU patients in the hospital crying out in pain. They became a haunting background noise and kept my nerves on heightened remembrance that this new reality was, in fact, real. Ambulance sirens wailed nonstop. Helicopters constantly landed on the roof of the hospital like a war zone. Hospital announcements any time of night or day paging this doctor or that doctor jolted our bodies up. Shift changes of faces coming and going left us no chance of becoming too dependent or familiar with any caregiver. It was like waking up repeatedly to a bad dream. Time slowed down for us in the hospital to the cadence of the IV drip.

Beep. Beep. Beep. Beep. The rhythmic methodical pacing of Anthony's lung machine was as hypnotic as it was unnerving. I am strong but, don't get me wrong, my nerves were wracked. I knew nothing, absolutely nothing, about spinal cord injuries (SCI). I could barely see clearly past the first night of the accident. It would be three months before I even realized what SCI meant. I was absolutely clueless.

Beep. Beep. Beep. SCREECH. SCREECH. SCREECH. The machine would set off a fire alarm emergency squeal. At the sound of the screaming machines, I rounded up nurses from down the hallway. Nurses never seemed to move fast enough for my comfort. Anthony's lungs were continuously filling up with fluid. He wouldn't be able to breathe as his body was struggling to get enough oxygen. During Anthony's stay at the hospital, he went through seven rounds of lung pumping to clear his lungs of water and allow him to breathe on his own. I jumped to the rafters of the ceiling every time that machine's warning noise went off, sending me in a near heart attack.

Additionally, because of the the amount of water consumed

by Anthony's body during his diving accident, he earned the title of having the most lung collapses, the opposite of his already constant lung compromises, in the history of Jackson Memorial Hospital. The space between his chest and his lung would fill with too much air and the doctors would have to re-inflate the lung. It's a lot to bear for any parent to watch the see-saw effects on their child like this, and I was not immune. Of all his trophies in his athletic life, this is one that neither he, nor I, could have ever seen in his fortune cards.

I am his mother. I am a strong woman. I am by personality naturally strong, but I had no idea just how hard my strength and faith in God were soon to be tested. However, my fright was bubbling inside me. Anthony was hooked up to all sorts of machines. I made known to the hospital staff Anthony's wishes to limit his medication to only what was necessary. Medication is something Anthony has continually refused following the initial injury. In the hospital, I had to stay strong and advocate for him.

I barked at hospital staff in protection of my son as they kept urging him, "He's not going to take anything."

Horror stories echoed in my head over and over of so many kids in situations like this - getting hooked on opioids because they were prescribed pain killers and the outcome ended up worse than the injury itself. I would see to it that it would not happen to Anthony. He was in pain, but the pain from the accident and surgery would go away. Being addicted to opioids could put Anthony in pain for far longer.

I also refused to let anyone say around Anthony and me: *paralyzed, paralysis, quadriplegic, handicapped, will never walk again.* There were times I threw doctors out of the room. I screamed at nurses if I felt it was necessary to get their attention. No one was going to tell me my son was going to be a vegetable. I knew I had to take some charge.

Winning the congeniality award or being popular at the hospital was not what I was concerned about. What I was concerned about was the well-being of my son. When I approached the nurse's station, they scampered away like mice. I didn't want to be the mean mom in the hospital, but being nice didn't get Anthony the help that was required for his level of injury.

I remember one nice mother, who sat patiently in the ICU reception, waiting two days for a doctor, a nurse, or anyone at the hospital, to give her an update on her son. Two Days!

After passing this patient lady for the fiftieth time, I asked her, "How long have they kept you waiting?"

She answered, "It's been two days."

In my head I throttled the head nurse like a PEZ dispenser. However, I loudly demanded directly to her, "You get this mother some answers."

Click. Click. Click. Click. The soft noise that had me jumping off my visitor seat in Anthony's room like Pavlov's dog was the clicking sound that came directly from Anthony. This was the sound Anthony would make with his tongue when he wanted my attention.

Click. Click. Click. Click. I would jump and quickly ask, "Anthony, what do you need?"

Following the accident, Anthony had temporarily lost his ability to talk. Amongst the tubes and machines, Anthony now had a feeding tube as a result of a tracheostomy. We created a communication system where he would not need to speak. We had a white dry-erase board with the twenty-six letters of the alphabet laid out and used a system similar to the Wheel of Fortune game show. I would move a marker slowly from A to Z and Anthony would, ever so slightly, blink his eyes when I hit the letter he wanted next to patiently form his words. In the timelessness of indefinite infinity, in a world that didn't exist outside the four walls of his hospital room, I would move the marker one letter at a time across the board in our new, and only, method of communication for about a month.

One morning, during my Wheel of Fortune communication game with Anthony, I asked, "A-n-g-e-? Angels? Anthony, were there angels?"

He would reveal to me that three angels were with him during his operation. In a *good way*, I was choosing to take this as a sign that things would get better. Our sign of hope.

Simultaneously, confirmed by the girls of the family — my nieces and daughter — they had a similar experience with angels surrounding Anthony. The girls had suddenly burst into tears right in the bathroom at the hospital when they heard Anthony's favorite song, "As Angels Cry" by Corey Smith, playing through the ceiling speaker in the bathroom. The day, the moment they heard it, also happened to be during Anthony's one, and only, life-saving surgery.

During this time, faith and family continued to surround Anthony. Mother Mary's statue arrived, as sent by my sister Terry, and was placed in a corner of his ICU room. Holy water was doused everywhere by my nieces.

When Anthony was later moved to his recovery room, it looked like the Sisters of the Sistine Chapel had visited by the time our entire family moved through it. Prayer circles were forming for Anthony inside and outside the hospital by everyone who was learning about his accident. As Anthony was confined to his bed, the familiar faces, well-wishes, and sacred trinkets gave him hope and comfort as he worked through the shock of his predicament. At the very least, it made family and friends feel better to surround Anthony with hope and love at all times.

I spent every morning in the hospital chapel for mass right after the doctors completed their rounds. When they asked for the prayer of our loved ones, I stood and said the same thing out loud every day, "May Anthony have a full recovery and walk again." I never missed hospital Mass.

Joe, Anthony's father, was right alongside me. He was instrumental in getting Frannie and me those last two seats on the flight to Florida the day of the accident. Even following our divorce, Joe and I have successfully run the family-owned-and-operated Global Cash Card company for years. I was doing board-level C-Suite presentations for our growing company when this accident happened to Anthony.

Joe and I were completely impenetrable in our commitment, devotion, and love on behalf of our son. We're complete opposites in how we handle these types of hard moments. Joe goes inward, and I stay outward. But here, together, we held hands in unified vigilance for Anthony. This is something I don't always see among the parents or those in relationships, but it is important and necessary for the recovery for someone with SCI.

Joe and I both took up residency at the hotel across the street during these ICU days. I mostly went there just to shower and nap when all the guests had to be out of the patient's room. We tag-teamed bedside vigils in between bathroom breaks, never leaving Anthony's side. Joe and I were in Anthony's room by 6 am every single morning when the doctors started their morning rounds. I had a journal and made notes about everything: what doctors came in, what nurses went out, what each doctor said, what each nurse did, Anthony's vitals, Anthony's movements, Anthony's progress, and Anthony's digress. Sometimes it's difficult to see progress when you're in the action, but after just one month, through my notes, I could see that Anthony was progressing. The first thing Anthony regained was his ability to speak. What a small thing we take for granted but a glorious start to recovery.

Additional visitors could come in to see Anthony, but only when either Joe or I stepped out of the room to surrender to the two visitors per patient hospital rule. One of us, either Joe or I, was always with Anthony. This was our personal parent rule. So many family and friends took shifts in the large reception area of Jackson Memorial that it became a sort of base camp, or communication hub, for these never-ending ICU days. You don't realize how long a day can become until you are doing literally nothing, except praying, each day for a month.

Our out-of-town family, like Anthony's older half brothers Joseph and Michael, flew in on the day of the accident and wore, day in and day out, the very few clothes they packed. Each family group took turns washing and camping in Jennifer and Matt's three bedroom Lighthouse Point, Florida home that was gratefully only forty-five minutes from the hospital. At least ten family members took up bunking there.

While Anthony ate from a feeding tube in his stomach those first few weeks, our main staple of food was chocolate chip cookies baked at night at Jennifer's and Matt's, and we carried out Au Bon Pain from the lobby of the hospital for breakfast, lunch, and dinner. To this day, I haven't been able to walk into another Au Bon Pain because of the reminder of those thirty days. Our lives as we knew had come to a complete halt.

Waves of silence would come and go. A few people might play cards to pass the time. Others dallied on their cell phones. A few took outside calls, and others listened to music through their headphones. Sometimes the background noise of the reception television droned on endlessly.

Then, like a standing wave of the crowd in a stadium, emotions come out like floods of tears and sobs of grief moving through the reception room of our family and friends, as the reality of the new reality begins to sink in. The shock of the severity of Anthony's spinal cord injury settled upon each of us in light of his shining life potential. Unified in his healing, all of us stayed. Anthony was living. Anthony was healing. But Anthony still did not have the ability to move. He still had a fight to enjoy his life. This was not what he wanted, and every time we saw him and could not help his body to do what it wanted, we re-experienced heartbreak.

Sometimes, to break the tension, the family went to the pub.

On the rare occasion Joe and I met up with our family, I emotionally would break down in the bar.

Sobbing, I asked, "How could this happen to Anthony?"

Having held it all together, mostly in front of Anthony, I simply lost it at times. One beer and I would cry like a baby. My niece, Tonya, hugged me as I felt my legs wanting to give out again. The shock, the grief, the loss, the confusion, the bargaining with God, the thanking God, the anger toward God...all of it.

With every ounce of my strength, I held it together so stoically for Anthony in the hospital. But out of the hospital, in a random environment like a bar, I would just fall apart. From my seat, and my soul, I cried. I cried for Anthony. When I cried for my son, my family circled up around me. This helped me to stay strong in front of, and for, Anthony.

What happened to Anthony could happen to anyone. I now always say *Anyone can slip on a banana peel and end up paralyzed.* According to the National Spinal Cord Injury Statistical Center (in 2019), between 249,000 and 363,000 Americans were estimated to be living with a spinal cord injury.[1] I would estimate that many of these SCI victims are worse off than they need to be. It affects the entire family, holding each caregiver hostage to another human being for survival at every moment.

There are two types of spinal cord injuries. There is a complete injury and incomplete injury. A complete spinal cord injury means there is no function below the level of the injury including no sensation and no voluntary movement. An incomplete spinal cord injury means there is some function below the primary level of injury.[2]

The complete injury affects function. For example, what is called an anterior cord syndrome is damage to the front of the spinal cord. This causes damage to the motor and sensory pathways

---

1 Data Source: Lasfargues JE, Custis D, Morrone F, Carswell J, Nguyen T. A model for estimating spinal cord injury prevalence in the United States. Paraplegia. 1995;33(2):62-68.
2 https://www.shepherd.org/patient-programs/spinal-cord-injury/about

of the spinal cord. Often, the victim struggles with movements but may retain some sensation. Anthony had no sensation following his accident and very limited movement.

Then there is damage to the center of the spinal cord known as central cord syndrome. The damage here includes the nerves that carry the signals from the brain to the spinal cord. The paralysis that happens here are loss of motor skills, paralysis in the arms, and partial impairment in the legs are common. Then there is the Brown-Sequard syndrome, which is damage to one side of the spinal cord.[3]

The higher up the cervical spinal cord injury is, the more severe symptoms will likely be. Anthony's accident involved his C5 and C6 vertebrae, known as a bruised spinal cord injury. His doctor said this was the worst case he had seen. Bruised is such a soft word given the severity of the damage and consequences.

Starting from the base of the skull with C1, count down four and five vertebrae from the top of your spine. This is the location of Anthony's injury. Touching your fingers down the back of your own neck, it would be right in the middle of the neck spine. Anthony lost all functions, both motor skills and sensory functions. He was considered C Level, an incomplete injury.

In comparison, Christopher Reeve, probably the most famous spinal cord injury victim of our time, suffered a C1 complete spinal cord injury. The C1, where Christopher Reeve severed, is the top of the spinal cord in the brain stem or atlas. This is the worst kind and elevated a level beyond Anthony's injury. Knowing what I know now about spine injuries, I'm surprised Christopher Reeve lasted as long as he did.

With 12,000 new injuries a year, being the loved-one of an SCI patient is like you are taking care of an infant, but it's actually worse. This is the best way I can describe the type of dependency I

---

3 https://www.aans.org/Patients/Neurosurgical-Conditions-and-Treatments/Spinal-Cord-Injury

witnessed through Anthony. Taking care of Anthony was like taking care of a twenty-three-year-old grown man who was incapacitated to the place of needing the type of care an infant requires.

Anthony was born weighing six pounds seven ounces. At the time of the injury, he weighed 175 pounds, but the weight loss from the physical atrophy began to show up almost immediately. Anthony needed someone to move him every two hours so he wouldn't get bed sores. Just another thing we had to worry about! This lasted for months after his injury. Not until we hit our next stage of healing did Anthony begin to make real progress.

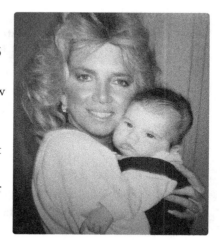

There is nothing a complete injury person can do for himself. They have full mental capacity trapped in a broken, unresponsive, non-functioning body. I could see Anthony through his eyes. He knew everything that was happening yet couldn't get his own body to listen to him and move that entire first month in the hospital.

The caregiver has to perform for their loved-one every single function that the body should do on its own. And it's not a caregiver that shows up for just two hours a day. Often the patient at this level of injury needs to be catheterized by the caregiver, given suppositories, bathed, dressed, and physically moved regularly just to keep bodily functions functioning. If this isn't done, the victim's organs will shut down and the person will die. Hear me. Not that the person can die, but will die. An unnecessary death that does not need to happen.

Again, since insurance doesn't cover this horrific injury, I ask, what do other families do who don't have the support, financial resources, volume of family members that Anthony has? At the end of the day, much of Anthony's primary care came right down to, simply, Joe and me. We would continue to spend the next seven years of our lives by Anthony's side ensuring that he would heal mentally and physically, and would continue to grow spiritually.

———◆———

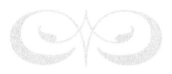

Jeremiah 29:11

"For I know the plans I have for you, says the Lord, plans for welfare and not for evil, to give you a future and a hope."

CHAPTER THREE

A False Hope

I t's the little wins that become remarkable milestones. In the ICU, the first milestone was that Anthony didn't die. He was stabilized but it was still touch and go. In the first forty-eight hours, this was obviously our biggest win.

After thirty days in the ICU, Anthony was transferred to rehab, still within Jackson Memorial Hospital. This sounds impressive. It's really not. Rehab is lame. It's too traditional.

I understand that hospitals do the best that they can with what they have regarding their budget, personnel, and available equipment. However, it can also be said that most hospitals do not specialize in the aftermath of paralysis, which is to the detriment of patients. Anthony was assigned three nurses, Cheryl, Lulu, and Sonia, during his stay at the hospital. They handled everything from feeding him, bathing him, flipping his body, shaving him to managing his everyday bodily functions. Sonia was always in high spirits and kept the mood light around Anthony. Anthony had to be continuously moved so that he did not develop bed sores or die. These ladies were dynamite and performed all of Anthony's bodily function tasks for him, things which we take for granted. I witnessed these ladies work with Anthony guided by patience, strength, and kindness, and he formed strong and intimate bonds with them within the rehab. The impact Lulu and Cheryl made on our family was lifelong, and today they continue to be Facebook friends. Lulu and Cheryl took really good care of him in rehab, and I am eternally grateful. I was not ready, nor prepared, for the task I was about to take head-on.

An occupational therapist named Maria and physical therapist named Mike, helped with things such as teaching Anthony to use his fork, since he was still unable to use his arms and hands. Marie would tie an Ace bandage to Anthony's hand with a fork tucked in the wrapping to give his body the sensation of movement; however, it was clumsy to witness. Mike helped with things like stretching his legs and moving his body, helping with blood circulation and muscle strengthening. Watching them was a small vision of what I could expect in my coming future to help Anthony in his healing journey.

Joe and I watched closely as Anthony would be placed on a full-size body board and strapped tightly to it. Then, slowly, the board would be propped upright with Anthony attached. These moments were simply glorious for us to witness. It was another milestone. I was so excited just to see Anthony, even with no strength of his own, vertical and upright. The purpose of this board was so circulation and blood flow would move through Anthony's system to prevent more atrophy. Anthony did not view the milestone in the same way I did.

To see him upright was like a brilliant memory of Anthony before the accident, as the tall and handsome man that he is. Of course, the reality was thinly veiled, as no part of him could be upright on his own. These were still big steps forward in my eyes. They represented hope, but he knew he still had so much more in front of him. Blood pressure is low for spinal cord injury patients, so any opportunity to be upright is important for the overall well-being of the body. This allows for things like flushing the lymphatic system and helping the heart with its circulation.

Every milestone was a victory, and even witnessing Anthony breathe in fresh air was such a big deal for all of us. Anthony's first shower since the accident was another milestone. These things happened slowly over the infinite time that existed in rehab. A milestone this week, another milestone that week, then another two weeks later. Anthony's body was going to heal and relearn at its own pace, no matter how much we wanted to rush the process.

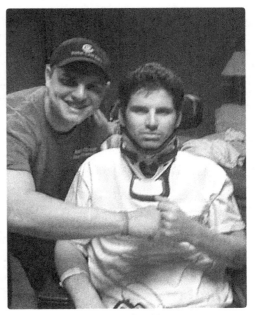

His cousin Joey shaved him while he was in rehab. Joey would come every day after football practice direct-ly to the hospital to be with Anthony. I know this sounds crazy, but I was just hit in fits of joy at seeing Anthony being shaved by Joey. The intimacy and brotherhood of support still gets me choked up when I think about it.

Tommy and Anthony

Every day, we were told the tracheotomy was going to be taken out. Then, it was not ready to come out. Another day, another false hope. It was heartbreaking to see Anthony's hopes dashed on a continuous basis. But then, one day it did come out! It finally came out and it was the biggest deal. Another huge mile-stone on our journey.

Anthony's cousin Tommy gave him his first sip of beer in rehab after the tracheotomy was removed. Anthony couldn't hold it up, but he took a sip, and that was pretty cool to see. It was a celebration, a toast in a way, of Anthony's survival.

Every day, Joe and I were with Anthony in rehab. Tommy and Kyle never left me sleeping alone at night. If Joe couldn't stay, one of those boys always slept on the hard couch in Anthony's room with me. I stayed by Anthony's side day in and day out. This was a very difficult time for Anthony, and he needed to see that no matter how long he needed us next to him, we were there when he went to sleep and when he would wake up.

After one month in rehab on a random morning, I was tapped on the shoulder by a nurse, "Today is your last day."

WHAAAAT??????

I had no clue what she was talking about. Anthony was still sleeping in his bed. I could hear the doctors who hadn't yet started their rounds.

It struck me... Then it struck me hard. Blown away.

Dispassionately, this unfamiliar nurse continued, "He's going to be discharged tomorrow."

We were given no other warning. No... anything. *And then they come and say it to me like that?* My mind began racing. Everybody in this hospital knew who I was. I was living there with Anthony for months; they saw me as much as they saw him. This was the first time that I learned Anthony was going to be discharged. I had zero ramp up or prep time to even consider taking Anthony home.

This was a big deal for us. This is a big deal for all families. This isn't like taking your newborn baby home from the hospital, and all mothers know what a displacing, yet exciting, feeling that can be. Mothers have an idea of what to expect and hopefully they've started preparing before the big day.

I charged firmly right down to the finance office. I expected more from the people who knew Anthony and me, who saw me every day, and who watched our slow progress. I never received discharge papers ahead of time nor was I made aware of a calendar end date for Anthony's discharge.

"This, 'Oh, by the way, your son is going home tomorrow,' is **NOT OKAY** by me," echoed through the four walls of the finance office upon deaf ears and complacent faces.

I was involved in every moment with Anthony every day, but I wasn't prepared to take him home. I wasn't a nurse like Lulu or Cheryl or a caregiver, and I hadn't planned for a Lulu or Cheryl type person to be scheduled at our house. Most importantly and above all else, Anthony was *definitely* not ready to come home.

That's what many hospitals do; they send people home in the blink of an eye. They kick them to the curb regardless of when they are ready or prepared.

"Yes, Mrs. Purcell, your insurance has run out."

Not to boast, but we have the best insurance money can buy. We could afford to be at the hospital. We were even already paying extra for him to be in a private rehab room. A small luxury that I am grateful I could give him.

"What do you mean our insurance has run out?" I stammered through with shock.

"I'm sorry. You've reached the maximum of coverage for rehab for spinal cord injury that the insurance company covers," stated the uncompassionate administrator.

"And I am just learning this today?" I quipped on my proverbial heel.

I stormed back upstairs to rehab and knew Joe was going to be writing a check to extend Anthony's stay.

"We can't take Anthony home yet. He's not ready. I'm not ready. But mostly, he's not ready, Joe!" I had to cover my hysterics in front of our son. I didn't want him any more nervous than me for his return home.

Joe wrote an outrageous check in the size of a yearly salary to the hospital, right on the spot, to extend Anthony's stay in rehab for thirty more days. A luxury, I'm aware, most families can't afford. I then went into overtime to do what I do, which was to seek out the best post-hospital spinal cord rehab possible in the world for my son.

I found Project Walk in Carlsbad, Southern California, which looked like Anthony's best hope. I called them right away and explained our situation and that Anthony still had very limited body control. We needed to go to them as soon as possible, especially since we no longer had the hospital support. At this particular moment, I received bad news.

"Sorry, Mrs. Purcell, we're fully booked with a two-month waiting list."

Is there a *good way* or a *bad way* to see this?

I was ready to negotiate and advocate for Anthony any way I could. "Get your owner on the phone with me right now."

Through my conviction, tenacity, and circumstances, I talked the owner, Ted Dardzinski, into finding space for Anthony.

We only stayed one additional week, of our pre-paid month, in our extended rehab at Jackson Memorial with no refund issued back.

The day came to leave the hospital that had been home for the past several months. In the morning, Anthony was strapped onto a board, and from the board, he slid into the discharge chair which is just a wheelchair. This wheelchair was different from the electric wheelchair he was using in rehab. It's the standard insurance liability wheelchair that patients are required to be pushed out of a hospital in so that no one slips and falls, breaks their neck, and more importantly, sues the hospital. The irony I felt as we were leaving.

Looking back years later, the best milestone was getting Anthony out of the hospital. After a lot of research and through our experiences, I found out that the quicker an SCI patient gets into aggressive focused rehab the quicker their recovery will be. If I kept him at Jackson Memorial Hospital, he wouldn't be nearly as mobile as he is today. The conventional rehab in hospitals… *it's baby shit.* They are not well-equipped, and the therapists are not specialized in spinal cord injury rehab.

Anthony's best day was also his worst day, notwithstanding the accident of course. There I was, waiting for Joe to bring the car around while looking at Anthony limp in a wheelchair wondering, *What now?* He couldn't walk, and he couldn't move his arms.

I felt like I was in a complete fog while Anthony sat strapped and limp in the wheelchair. I stared right into Anthony's eyes. He had no strength, either in his body or his spirit. He had on a neck brace which propped his flopped head up. He was kind of like a baby, but worse. Yet, here we were together, leaving the hospital for the abyss.

I remember thinking about Joe driving around to pick me up with Anthony in my arms as a newborn while I was the one who sat in the proverbial don't slip and fall and sue wheelchair. I remember holding both my babies, Anthony and Jennifer, after birth while waiting for Joe to come with the car, but this was very different. Very wrong. There are plenty of rule books for knowing what you are going to do as a new mother, but there was absolutely no rule book going home with me now. I had been so in the moment in the hospital that I didn't even think about this chapter of our journey.

Ironically, we had just moved out of a townhouse that was full of stairs which had now become the mortal enemy of Anthony's life. Stairs are the arch enemy to any spinal cord injury victim.

Instead, we were going home to this newly decorated fresh condo, and it was exactly as it had always been yet it was completely different…completely unfitting. For the first time, since the accident, I was home alone with Anthony. Absolute deafening silence after weeks of absolute noise.

Silence.

His door was closed. He had full and complete privacy. There was no hope that day in him when we arrived home. Throughout the echoes of the house, his sobs started. There I was standing in the skeletal bones of a life we both once knew that no longer would serve us going forward. There was nothing here for us, but really, there was nothing here for Anthony.

Alone. All alone.

Not only was he coming to terms with being trapped in his body, his bedroom was like being trapped in a life that was a trophy. We had just completed mounting a large fish from one of his big fishing trips. Anthony loved the water and fishing was an extension of that love. In addition, his walls were covered with photos, trophies, and medals from his JV and Varsity sport teams. Pictures of him as a model. Nothing in his room could he reach for, nothing in his room could he touch or be again, both physically or metaphorically. He was in the mausoleum of a life that was now dead. Everything that covered the walls and his space was no longer accessible to him in his life now. I didn't have time to change it. And I didn't know how to change it.

I couldn't imagine his pain. Not his physical pain. We were well beyond that. Instead, his heartache. This young man, twenty-three years old, with the world in the palm of his hand — good looking, educated, athletic, up and coming, a ladies man — now trapped in his body that was no longer of his own command.

Listening to Anthony's cry was painful. When I tell you it was painful, it means I could have thrown up. This was one of the most painful moments of my life. As I said, when your kid is happy, you are happy, and when your kid's soul hurts, your soul throbs in pain too. It was horrible. I knew, as his mother, he had to cry it out.

Sell your books at
Go to sellbackyourBook.com
and get an instant price quote.
We even pay the shipping - see
what your old books are worth
today!

I wasn't going to let him quit on himself. I would let him cry... tonight.

This type of injury is as much mental as it is physical. I would let him have his pain tonight even if to the shudder of my own fears, but I wasn't going to let him die inside himself or let him not live his life to his fullest potential. No. I wasn't. Not Anthony. No way. Tomorrow was a new day for both of us.

———•—

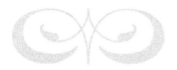

Psalm 46:10

*"Be still and know that
I am God."*

CHAPTER FOUR

Bite Off More Than You Can Chew and Chew Like Hell!

ven though Anthony and Tommy are literally cousins, they are more like brothers. They grew up together and were inseparable. They had a personal falling out right before the accident and were not speaking at the time that Anthony injured himself. It was the kind of rift that made the entire family feel uncomfortable.

Tommy, who had been attending Florida State University, dropped everything, including school, to be by Anthony's side. Tommy happens to be a big guy and was strong enough to lift Anthony up and down. Up and down. Stretched. Moved. Transferred. Carried. Wheelchairs. Beds. Cars. Crazy. Lifesaving to Anthony and me. I knew I could count on Tommy to do the literal heavy lifting where I couldn't, as Anthony still did not have control of any of his body.

After Anthony spent the night crying, I woke up ready to lift his spirits. This day was the first step toward Anthony's real physical recovery. Tommy did what he would do for Anthony and lifted him up, and put Anthony into the wheelchair. We called for a van, and Joe chartered a private jet for the four of us to travel to Project Walk in California.

Well-meaning and well-intended neighbors gathered around us like they were looking at a unicorn. They were trying to smile kindly. However, what I saw was more along the lines of shock and pity. Some approached slowly to hug, and we let them. Having come off the grief of the night before, I was so incredibly sensitive and uncomfortable with what Anthony must have been feeling as he was stared at by everyone in a crowd. And worse, he couldn't do anything. He couldn't hug them back. He was just quiet.

"Thank you for your well wishes. Anthony is going to be just fine." I repeated to everyone who came up to us. This wasn't for me but for Anthony; I was selling *my good way* of looking at things for the sake of the staring neighbors and awkward well-wishers.

"We appreciate all of your prayers. Thank you." I said cheerily and loudly to people standing about us, as though to really say to them, *Look away. Mind your business.*

The humiliation!

Even though every single one of these neighbors came with good intentions, and I know they cared about us, Anthony and I had no energy to speak or even to hear from them. Not in this *still* raw moment for us. It was an absolute humiliation for Anthony, but I couldn't dwell on this moment with him. I knew we had a flight to board and a rehab center waiting for us in Carlsbad, California, north of San Diego, and just south of the well-known military base Camp Pendleton. We had an unknown life ahead of us, and a dead one to leave behind.

On the west coast, we made sure to settle into an easy handicap accessible one-floor living space to accommodate Anthony at the

Pelican Villas in Newport Beach, California. We chose Newport because Joe and our family business was located there, and it was a pretty straight drive to Carlsbad.

Anthony would start intensive physical therapy three hours a day, three days a week. I persuaded Ted, the owner of Project Walk, to personally train Anthony, as I knew he was the best bet for Anthony to recover. I shared with Ted the severity of what I had researched and was ready to roll up my own sleeves to pitch

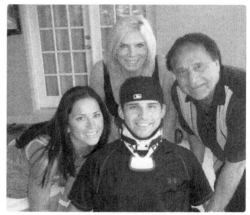

Jennifer, Micki, Anthony, and Joe

in where needed and necessary. I was right. Ted got Anthony off and running quickly, pardon my pun.

I made sure to communicate with everyone associated with Project Walk. The owner. The trainers. The support staff. The other families. The victims. This is what I do. I would get to know them and what they were also trying to achieve. My son was going to get the best care and be surrounded by people who all cheered for each other.

Ted and I eventually became good friends. I got so involved in Project Walk that I would eventually MC their annual events where they celebrated their latest successful SCI clients who could walk the red carpet. We would all scream with joy like our lives depended upon it in celebration of the victory for the success of the clients.

At night, Anthony had panic attacks, realizing again he was trapped inside his body. Although progress was good at Project Walk, it was slow. This meant it was slow progress just to move fingers. It was recommended that he take Xanax for his anxiety by his overseeing doctor. The pressure to take the medication was fierce and practically relentless from everyone involved in health and body.

Anthony didn't want it, and I agreed with Anthony to not take it. I kept encouraging Anthony to stay strong, he could get through all this.

From our rented place at the Pelican, we began to settle in. During the week, Joe and I set an alarm every two hours taking shifts to roll Anthony in his bed so that he wouldn't get bedsores. This was what the hospital left us to deal with.

On the weekend, I did this two-hour drill, no matter what, all by myself. I had to become Lulu and Cheryl, a role I never dreamed of, but one that I owned like my life depended on it, a role that I owned as if my son's life did depend on it. I would tend to the many needs Anthony now had for all of his bodily functions to work and not break down.

It took me about two to three weeks to work our new caregiver, Norma, into the mix of this mess. She began handling his everyday tasks, which gave me some relief. To this day, Anthony still has Norma, who has stayed by his side from the very beginning of his journey in California.

The enthusiasm for Project Walk was infectious to us, except for Anthony who was jaded. It was a big part of the culture at Project Walk to tell victims that they will walk again. Anthony hated, and still does hate, being told that he is going to walk again. It's a *bullshit* thing to say. From experience, don't say it. Don't say it to Spinal Cord Injury victims because you don't know if they will be able to walk again. Even as far as Anthony has come, to this day, he still cannot walk. Today, he can wear a brace to stand in place, kinda. Now, as his mother, his cheerleader, and his advocate, in *my good way of looking at things* I'm not giving up. But still, we don't know. We just keep pushing forward one day at a time. And it's a long and difficult journey.

It was during this time at Project Walk that I recognized the important need of rehabilitation for spinal cord injury victims. Slowly, I began to see Anthony gain control of his neck, then came his hands,

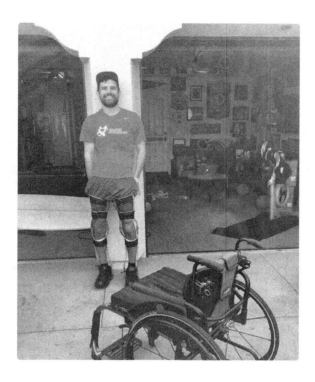

and his arms. He gained upper body strength. This was our slow and painful process. It was a daily commitment by Anthony and I. We learned stretches, weight routines, and of course, we had to keep Anthony's spirits up through all of this. We learned to use certain machines that could keep Anthony's body in motion and move him in ways that he didn't have control of.

During Anthony's healing process, I became aware that this intense physical form of treatment was not accessible to most who needed it. Joe and I built up an enormous family business, and through this we were able to give Anthony everything he needed and still needs for his healing journey. This has cost us outrageous amounts of money that some people may not be fortunate enough to see in their lifetime. Additionally, I was able to be with Anthony every single day, in what became our journey, because of the success we had built in business.

But I understand most people may not be able to do the same

for their own family. As I looked around from my own situation with Anthony, I truly began to see what other families were dealing with, and it broke my heart.

One kid came in with a jar full of coins just to use the functional electrical stimulation bike, or FES bike, at Project Walk. These bikes are popular amongst the spinal cord community because it allows someone with little to no voluntary leg movement to pedal a stationary bike through electrodes that stimulate the muscles to contract and motion automatically. It is vital for recovery for spinal cord victims. I watched this kid come in with his jar of coins to cover the FES bike costs of $25.00 an hour to get his ride in.

While I was at Project Walk, I saw another parent and heard his story. He was a father who drove his kid thousands of miles across country specifically to Project Walk to beg them to take his sixteen-year-old son. Frankly, I understood this father's desperation, because I did this very same thing. Except Project Walk didn't take the man's son. They were turned away due to lack of funds to cover the $100.00 an hour rehab fees. His son was lying in the backseat and couldn't even sit up.

I knew this man's pain. I had that pain too when they first told me that they couldn't help us due to space restrictions, until I was able to negotiate having Anthony there. What would I have done if I couldn't get Anthony in? This is what spinal cord injury victims have to think about and go through. I kept thinking, *This isn't right.* If Project Walk couldn't help them, then who was helping people who may not have the connections or the means for continuous physical therapy? My anxiety and discomfort around what I was witnessing increasingly grew.

As a business owner, I understand firsthand that you can't stay in business if you let everyone drain your resources. You have overhead for the space, the equipment, the staffing, the insurance, the taxes, but *My God!* I still couldn't believe what I was witnessing. Since I was there all the time, I talked with the trainers and with the families. I heard the problems, the issues, and the limitations. But the consequence of not getting this physical help is more disastrous than most people may understand. The tools and equipment and help can be the difference between a good life and a bad life — and sometimes the difference of having a life at all. Someone had to help these people. Clearly, God put me next to Anthony so we could make a change. Family and faith in God is everything to me.

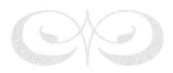

Philippians 4:13

"I can do all things through Christ who strengthens me."

CHAPTER FIVE

Suicide

Six months after Anthony and I returned home from the hospital, and through his intense and continuous physical sessions with Project Walk in our new life in California, he had gained back some control over his own body. It still wasn't full control by any means, but he could fully speak, move his arms, though not very high, and control his neck and head. He could also type, albeit slowly, as full extension of his fingers and quickness were no match to what they used to be.

Six months out of the hospital, with all the successes and the encouragement by others and myself, I walked in on him researching suicide online. This moment with Anthony was almost as horrifying as the news of the accident itself. He was sitting in bed with his laptop open in front of him. I could feel my pulse pounding as I looked over his shoulder and sharply asked, "Anthony, what are you doing?"

"I'm on suicide websites, and I want to check out," he replied, without so much as glancing up from the screen. "I want to die."

What?

This was a serious Red Alert moment. My son was plotting to kill himself. *Bullshit*, I thought. *My son is not going to die.* The accident didn't kill him, and I'm not going to let him kill himself either.

Panic inside me. I knew Anthony was depressed, and I even felt suspicious to the point where I felt on guard that this looming option could someday be considered by him. I'm not ignorant to why he would feel this way or why he would choose this way out of his situation. When Norma left every morning, I became an extension of Anthony's arms and legs at his beck and call for his every need. It was difficult for us both, but I knew I had to be strong. No matter what I went through, I knew he was suffering even more.

There had to be some way for me to show him his life still had value, that being paralyzed wasn't the end of the world, and that he still had something to offer, something to contribute, and was capable of making a powerful difference. Maybe he could even use his experiences and his pain to help others who weren't as fortunate as our family. I began to think of how many other Anthonys there were, and how many might not be able to access the help they needed. I cannot be the mom who just smiles and says, "It'll be alright." It's not the truth. There is always an action to take.

What is a good way *of looking at this?* I asked myself.

Taking a deep breath, I looked my discouraged, despondent son in the eye and said, "Anthony, we're going to start a charity."

"Fuck you," he quickly and bluntly replied angrily to me.

Figuratively hurled back by his pain thrown at me for a moment, I regained my inner balance. Knowing all along what he was going through, who could blame him for his feelings and his anger? But in our family, quitting isn't on the agenda. We choose to find the upside of every angle. I knew I needed to make my son mentally strong, to choose to see an upside in addition to the physical strength he was gaining, if he was going to survive and thrive following his accident. I knew if we started a charity it would help my son progress mentally every day, and give him something to live for. It would make him see outside his own pain and also know he was not alone.

Paralysis affected Anthony's body and it affected his mental state. His cognitive abilities were still in tact, but depression hit hard. The new life that he had to come to terms with was a very difficult transition. I had to climb into Anthony's head every single day to care for him in the way he needed outside of just making sure he moved his body. I had to climb into his head to keep him strong. Ultimately, this charity is what built Anthony's mental strength.

Our journey of Walking With Anthony wouldn't be an easy one. It wouldn't be easy for Anthony, and as I continuously pushed us forward, I left no room for it to be easy for me either. Fierce, furious, and undeterred, I looked forward because I wasn't about to lose my son to his despair. If he survived this tragic accident, I would make sure he would survive the aftermath.

Anthony had been prescribed hardcore depression medication to help deal with his anxiety and depression that hung over him like a cloud after the accident every single day. Still, Anthony refused this way out of his pain. I didn't want him to take the meds either, even as I knew we were confronting this nebulous dark fated moment. I knew he was depressed, but it was my job to keep him going and to build him back up to become happy and stable again. I knew I could push him to heal without the aid of prescriptions. It was a mental game now, and that was a game we could and would win together. Psychoactive drugs, in my opinion, were not his way out. The over-prescribing of these medications is a nationally reported crisis. We are aware of opioid addiction, and that was a battle we didn't want to add to our ever increasing difficulties.

I never asked Anthony about the details as to how he planned on committing suicide. My worst thought, of course, would be that he would overdose by doctor-prescribed medication. Fortunately, together we battled through his depression, and I never needed to dig deeper with him.

This crossroad is a real issue for SCI survivors. Many, if not most, spinal cord injury victims suffer from depression, anxiety, and PTSD as a result of their injuries. The aftermath can be as traumatic as the accident itself. Study after study shows that the risk of suicide is higher after a spinal cord injury than it is for the average able-bodied person.

It was obvious to me that surviving an accident into paralysis would lead to wanting to commit suicide. The accident was the sudden impact, like a tsunami hitting your life, your psyche, and your body first, and then about six months later, the second wave, the post-traumatic stress disorder, hits home as the victim has to come to terms with their new reality. Imagine all the goals that you have now, and then imagine they are taken from you in a split second, and you'd be left knowing that they could no longer come true in the way you imagined.

It's a tough life transition to find peace and acceptance for yourself. Unfortunately, some never do. The victims have to mourn the life they once lived. They have to mourn the life they now will never know. For Anthony, his mourning began the night he went to our home in Florida right after the hospital. He went home to a room full of trophies and photos and began grieving the life he thought he would have lived. I know this is not the life Anthony expected, but I also knew that while it might end up looking different, it could still be amazing! And that was a *good way* of looking at it. There will still be more to life for Anthony than what he may have thought for himself.

The social abandonment is as isolating as the paralysis and as debilitating as the mental despair that sets in following the accident. For the first year following Anthony's accident, he never left our villa except to go to Project Walk. He was ashamed to be seen in a wheelchair even if it was by complete strangers. He didn't want the reflection back of the pity he was already feeling for himself.

In the same way, as I fought for my son's physical rehab, I found myself fighting for his mental sanity through the idea of beginning a charity together, Walking With Anthony. The name hit me like lightning. I love my son's name, and I was walking with him, whether he always realized it or not, through all his ups and his many downs.

I also had to fight for his social life to stabilize. Most SCI victims are abandoned by their peers soon after the initial accident. It's painful to witness. It's awkward. What does someone say? How do you fake small talk amongst the inevitable truth of someone's life that had changed unexpectedly? It's hard, and both Anthony and I are aware of it.

You hear it all the time from caregivers and family—"What happened to all his friends? How come no one visits?" Part of it, I'm sure, is that people just don't know how to act. People don't know what to say.

I remember when my father was dying, my uncle just stopped coming when we all knew the end was near. He simply couldn't handle seeing his brother in that condition. People simply walk away when someone has this type of physical injury. It seems unbelievable, but it happens more than you can imagine. It's just a big part of the accident— you can't go out and play basketball, you can't do this, you can't do that—and eventually friends begin to just drift away. It's terribly sad, yet oddly understandable.

Honestly, I never truly considered what someone in a wheelchair had gone through or experienced before Anthony's own accident. Now, I go up to them all the time. I offer to buy them a beer and engage them in conversation. I always ask what happened and how they're coping. SCI victims do not lose their personality or their mental state with their mobility. I noticed that they tend to like to share their stories, but most people just sweep them under the rug and aren't open to listening. As I do with Anthony, I try to motivate them and give them hope and let them know that I see them. People are afraid to ask them anything and that's what is behind the awkwardness for most people...the avoidance comes off as pity.

Anthony, before the accident, was such a vibrant, athletic guy, and was always the leader of the group he was with. He was the ring-leader in all sorts of stuff, and when he got hurt, he was so fortunate that his friends and all his family stuck with him.

My brother Tommy took care of Anthony during the seventh and eighth grades while Joe and I were going through our divorce. Tommy took Anthony to many of his basketball games after school while I rushed over from work. Uncle Tommy played basketball with the boys in the driveway when he was done with his work. By ninth grade, Anthony already made varsity and just as easily made friends his own age, and earned the respect of his older teammates. Our re-frigerator was full of pictures as we posted Anthony's teams alongside his friends and his cousins.

What stands out, even to this day, is that Anthony's friends al-ways looked up to him as a leader. He is respected by his friends both in business and in friendship. His strongest friendships have never faltered even during his most difficult times. Everyone in the family constantly shows up and gives him support. The immediate after-math is always of the utmost importance. Anthony has twenty-eight cousins, and they were constantly sending him texts and emails. That's the kind of support all victims need but not all are fortunate to have. In spite of all this beautiful support, Anthony still isolated himself. Again, I was determined to walk with Anthony through his pain to help him feel like himself again.

Anthony's birthday has always been a big deal for him because it takes place on New Year's Eve. For his twenty-fourth birthday, just under a year after his accident, Joe rented a yacht out of Newport Beach, and I planned his party. Anthony thought it was just going to be a small family get together (no such thing as a small family for us), but I invited all of his friends and cousins from back home in Florida and our new home in Southern California as a big surprise to him. Anthony was relaxing on the yacht having a few beers and one by one each friend made a surprise entrance from the back of the boat. All of his buddies strutted out like it was no big deal, one after the other. He hadn't seen most of these guys since he was in the hospital rehab in Florida when he couldn't talk or shake their hand. This time, he could show his expression of happiness and gratitude.

When Boomer stepped out, all I could think about was how Boomer, Anthony's old high school friend, had thrown himself over Anthony and sobbed like a baby when he saw Anthony laid up in the hospital. Here, like all of Anthony's friends, Boomer stuck around. The tears were no longer sorrow but joy to be with each other and to celebrate Anthony.

Anthony was blown away by the party—he had no idea who'd be coming out next. I could tell his head was spinning—but it was exactly what he needed to lift his spirits and his soul. Seeing all of his friends who were there to support him and celebrate his life had a huge impact on him. It broke the isolation of his personal solitary confinement. It brought him out of his own head. He forgot about his bodily circumstances and simply enjoyed being just Anthony with his friends.

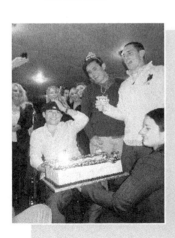
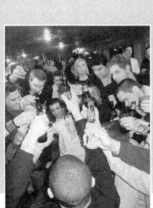
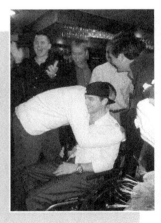

This is the way we need to treat our fellow SCI victims. We need to treat their body, their mind, and also their soul. Feeding their soul creates their will to live and keeps it burning inside of themselves. For Anthony, facing his twenty-fourth birthday was a real turnaround. To this day, now in his early thirties, his friends have stuck with him. He just recently took a trip to San Diego with twenty of his buddies for their NFL fantasy football draft. I was so happy to see them all together.

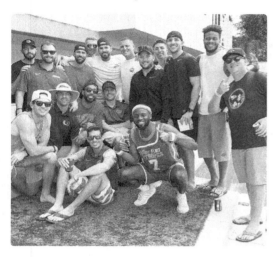

Blessed in our lives by abundance and God, Anthony's friends and family showed up when he needed them. Tommy played a huge role in keeping him mentally and physically pumped up. He dedicated all his spare time to keep Anthony company either by working out with him, visiting us while we were in Newport Beach for Anthony's recovery, and even driving him to Carlsbad to meet with trainers everyday. He has been a faithful and dedicated cousin in a way that kept Anthony feeling like his normal self before the accident. Tommy was relentless; he just kept kicking Anthony's ass to keep going, even when things seemed impossible. Cousin Kyle, whose brother is Bernie who saved Anthony when he was floating and limp in the ocean, also always came by to visit and keep Anthony company.

These two cousins, and his good friends Bill and Sean, fought hard to make sure Anthony's spirits were lifted and tried to keep him feeling the familiarity of life before, even with simple things like sharing a Bud Light with him. Anthony sometimes needed the tough love to keep pushing and striving forward. It couldn't always come from me. I had to have support too.

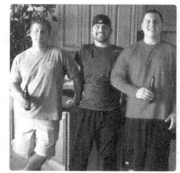

Sean, Anthony and Tommy

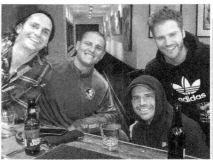

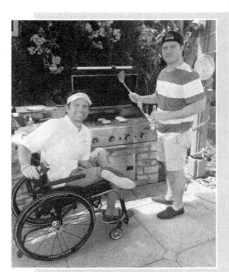

Bill, Tommy, Anthony and Kyle

Anthony and Kyle

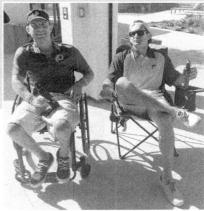

Anthony and Bill

It relieved me of full-time duties to my son to ensure I didn't get burnt out myself.

A car accident left Chris, a truly beautiful soul, paralyzed from the waist down when he was about to turn twenty-five years old. After a lifetime as an athlete and working in the family business, he suddenly found himself dependent on others. His medical bills bankrupted him and forced his single mother to sell most of everything they had to keep him alive. It got to the point of isolation that he didn't even want to move out of his bed.

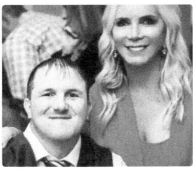

Micki and Chris

His mother, Cheryl, would call me, desperate, and say, "Micki, what do I do? He doesn't even want to get out of bed. His friends have stopped seeing him."

Cheryl just didn't have enough by herself. Not enough to give hope.

Not enough to give strength. Not enough to give comfort. Not enough to give him the type of care required to sustain the healthy and productive life he wanted and deserved.

When I received Cheryl's text one evening, reading only, *Chris died today*, I knew what had happened. It was while writing this book, that Chris, an SCI victim, overdosed on pain medication. It was suicide.

This happens all the time. How do you respond to a mother whose son overdoses after surviving an accident that leaves him paralyzed? It's an ironic quandary. He was only thirty-one, which means he survived six years after his accident. We had been rooting Chris on! This heartbreak is always so painful. It was painful for Chris. It is painful for his mother. Painful for all of us. Just like so many others before with spinal cord injuries, Chris died by overdosing on his prescription medication. I think about his poor mother. I think of Anthony, and if he had been taking prescription pain medication, would he have done the same when he considered suicide?

As I choke up to make the return phone call of unspeakable condolence to Cheryl, I reminded myself that we know this happens. It was the same neglect and lack of support that had caused so many other paralysis victims to take their own lives in despair. This unacceptable state of affairs continues to persist, and it needs to end. The families and loved ones of the disabled, as well as those that advocate for them, need so much more help and support than they receive. The depression, the pain, the anguish that spinal cord injury survivors go through is a reality. For Cheryl—a single mother without the time and resources to support her son in the way he needed—it was almost too much. As a mom, she did the best she could with the resources she had. She also wasn't the type of personality that would advocate loudly when needed to.

I do not blame Cheryl for the fact that Chris overdosed. Everyone involved is doing the best that they can with their circumstances. That is why my public plea is loud so people become aware of what an SCI victim goes through and how their life transitions.

Cheryl wasn't able to do the two-hour bed flip every day and every night for physical circulation that Chris's body required. She had to go to work. She had to work to keep his medical insurance in place. Chris's mother also didn't push him in the way that all SCI victims need to be pushed — in mind and spirit. Again, this is as much a mental game as it is a physical challenge. The isolation also needs to be broken.

Anthony had, and still has, the support that 99.9% of SCI victims don't seem to have because the people in their life abandon them. They don't know what to say to the victim, and then they wither away in the background until they disappear out of the victim's life. The social abandonment is real. It is isolating and it is equally devastating as a consequence of the accident itself. In Anthony's case, he did have social support from family and friends. I wanted to ensure Walking With Anthony would be a nonprofit that would offer friendships and real connections.

Christopher Reeve talked publicly about his desire to commit suicide after his accident. Famous for playing Superman in the 80s, and similar to Anthony in the looks and height department, Christopher Reeve was paralyzed from the neck down after a horse jumping accident and was looking for his way out of his tragic predicament. Left without the use of his arms and legs and unable to even breathe without mechanical assistance, Reeve found inspiration as a spokesman advocating for other people who can't call the president or a senator or testify before Congress about the real issues for disabled people.

Like Superman, I decided Anthony and I would start a foundation of our own and dedicate it to helping spinal cord injury survivors live their best lives. I was determined for Anthony and for every other victim struggling to regain their mobility and independence.

I had to think about what real impact we wanted to make. Unlike the Christopher Reeve foundation, where money goes into research, Walking With Anthony would directly help victims and families who couldn't afford rehab or specialized equipment. And most importantly, we would build a supportive, informed, and compassionate community for victims and their families.

Rehabilitation would be our major priority. It can easily cost $100 an hour, and as my family learned from bitter experience, even the best insurance doesn't come close to covering what's really necessary to heal. In fact, many people living with spinal cord injuries find themselves having to choose between paying for their therapy or paying their rent.

Caregiving is a huge undertaking for those with SCI. You and I take daily tasks such as getting out of bed, dressing, or even just daily hygiene tasks for granted. Someone with a spinal cord injury often needs someone to help with something as simple as brushing their teeth—and that kind of assistance doesn't come cheap. An experienced home health aide (HHA) can run as much as $65,000 a year or more! Then there's the cost of special equipment. Electric wheelchairs can cost nearly $30,000. A standing frame is $12,000, and this is something Anthony utilized often to keep his blood flow circulation in the beginning of his recovery. A customized bed could run at about $4,000. An FES bike, which electrically stimulates the leg muscles of a paraplegic, is another $18,000. Then we have the ongoing costs of basic supplies like catheters and urine drainage bags, adult diapers, sterile gloves, and other necessities to keep life going. There are too many to list, and it adds up quickly. And don't get me started on the cost of drugs. I'm not talking about light medication like over the counter Tylenol. I'm talking about heavy prescription medication for people with incredibly severe and deep depression.

All in all, the lifetime costs for someone living with SCI can be more than $4.5 million dollars. We're talking about money that most people simply do not have on hand. The vast majority of family bankruptcies—66.5% according to CNBC[4] —are due to medical expenses. *How hard must it be for those less fortunate than our family? How hard must it be for someone with NO family?* Those were my thoughts as I shared my ideas with my family and friends about Walking With

---

[4] https://www.aans.org/Patients/Neurosurgical-Conditions-and-Treatments/Spinal-Cord-Injury

Anthony. This led to my establishing an emergency fund as part of our charity, and the creation of a community where families and survivors could share resources and experiences, so they don't have to feel like they're facing such an enormous and life-changing crisis alone. No one plans to have a SCI, but the immediate financial and emotional costs in the wake of an accident are astronomical.

Understandably, my friends and family were protective of my time, energy, and resources. Everyone knew that taking care of Anthony had already become my life. No one wanted to see me expend extra *Micki* energy on a new venture or project. My life was full immersion into Anthony. I was ready for this challenge though, as I wanted to make a difference and knew it would be more than just a positive influence for Anthony, but for many others in similar situations like his.

"Micki, you have no idea what goes into a charity," said one dear friend who was highly involved in charity work. "It costs money to set up something like that, and you'll spend your whole time with the charity asking other people for money."

"Running a charity isn't like running a business, Micki," another well-intentioned friend lovingly warned. "You already have your hands full with Anthony and your businesses. You've barely been able to catch up on yourself since Anthony had his accident, how on earth will you find the time to run a foundation?"

My biggest critic of all, however, was Anthony.

"You're crazy, mom," he said with a tinge of bitterness to my resolve.

"You watch!" I told Anthony. "One of these days, you're going to thank me."

This charity needed to be a positive to keep Anthony alive. And if I could keep Anthony alive with this charity, how many other SCI victims could this charity keep alive and help thrive!

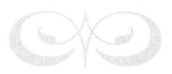

Isaiah 40:31

"But they who wait for the Lord shall renew their strength, they shall mount up with wings like eagles, they shall run and not be weary, they shall walk and not faint."

CHAPTER SIX

Baby Steps and Great Leaps Forward

It's simply underestimated how important regular exercise is for people with SCI. They're more likely to be overweight, with high cholesterol, and high blood pressure. This puts them at higher risk for cardiovascular and other diseases. In fact, for more than a decade, experts at the U.S. Department of Health and Human Services have recommended that paraplegics and quadriplegics get "at least 150 minutes per week of moderate-intensity aerobic exercise and two days per week of muscle-strengthening exercise."[5] SCI victims need to build up their muscle endurance by lighter and more repetitive weight training. On top of that, they also recommend nearly three hours of "vigorous" aerobic exercise every week, and even still on top of *that*, a recommendation of at least two days per week of strength training (slower, heavier weights). Together, this ensures every single muscle gets a workout that people without SCI normally

---

5 http://www.cdc.gov/physicalactivity/everyone/guidelines/

get just by walking. Think about that next time you have the opportunity to work out in the morning, and you think, "Ah, no! Not today." I have seen with my own eyes the tremendous results that are possible through exercise and strength training and even stretching. Stretching is a big part of the physical therapy rehab process because SCI victims are highly susceptible to stiff muscles and joints.

A study published in the *Journal of Spinal Cord Medicine* showed that physical therapy has positive effects, both physical and mental, on victims struggling with spinal cord injuries. I think building that positive mental attitude might be the most important part—as it is too easy to give up.

Equipment is expensive for spinal cord injury patients but is important for recovery. Gait trainers, which are large devices with wheels that someone with paralysis can use to help walk independently or relearn to walk again, are extremely useful. There are vibrating machines that force automatic muscle contractions that are required for the body. There are sling suspension exercises and standing machines. Until you're dealing with a spinal cord injury, you might have no idea items like these even existed, or especially how expensive they are.

FES bikes help with far more than just leg exercises; they also help with breathing, grasping, standing and walking, and even better bladder and bowel function. The physical therapy never seemed to end, but neither did the encouragement. We didn't know it at the time, but the encouragement wasn't just the therapists' goodwill. It was part and parcel of the program that we were participating in. This was meant to address Anthony's emotional health and build up the confidence he'd need to re-acquire some physical independence and to accept those things he might never be able to do again. He worked hard to regain the ability to use his arms again and to be able to control his bodily functions. Outside of his actual ability to walk, he has a lot of control of his bodily functions now.

Eventually, we hoped Anthony would be able to make use of some adaptive devices to help him with his daily activities, but we also knew it was going to be a long haul for everyone in our family. We tried everything to help aid his recovery outside the standard of care that was suggested. Massage. Acupuncture. We even tried stem cell therapy, which to this day Anthony doesn't really believe worked. I'm definitely not as doubtful. It's not like you swallow a handful of stem cells and suddenly you're running around and shooting baskets. It takes time and patience. I know the details of Anthony's condition better than anyone, and he has progressed more than just about anyone else I've seen at his level of injury.

Each injury is unique, but what I witnessed with Anthony was nothing short of miraculous. People didn't think he would move his hands and arms again. But his hands greatly improved. Many of his personal functions returned. There's no way to know for sure, of course, if it was directly related to stem cells, as he'll be rehabbing for the rest of his life; however, I am convinced that the stem cell therapy assisted him. It's difficult to pinpoint exactly because we were trying everything and "the kitchen sink" for Anthony's recovery. Rehab is non-negotiable for healing regardless of any other method of treatment.

Occupational therapists play a huge role in a spinal cord injury victim's rehabilitation, with the goal of helping the victims get their lives back. While the physical therapists were working on his legs and arms, the occupational therapists focused on Anthony's fine motor skills as well, so he could accomplish simple activities you and I take for granted, like using a knife and fork, dialing a phone, holding a pen or pencil, or typing on a computer. And they worked on some of the less sexy activities, like bladder and bowel control. This was actually really important for Anthony, a handsome guy who had always done well with the ladies. Being unable to control these most basic biological functions had been a source of embarrassment to him. Bekah Thorne also came in to give Anthony deep tissue massages weekly to help with his muscle tone and blood circulation. They became very close friends. As therapy went on and his spirits began to brighten with his improvement, Anthony began to grow more eager every day to manage his own life.

Project Walk worked wonders with Anthony in his first few months coming out of the hospital. However, while there, the founder retired and then we had to deal with a new management team that came in. They didn't display the same passion that the original team had, nor did they hold the same integrity. Anthony lost all his momentum and motivation to continue participating at Project Walk and we soon left.

Later it was revealed that the new team and Project Walk were shut down for misappropriation of funds. It was very disappointing, to say the least, not just for us, but for the many others that would never have the opportunity to get the help they needed.

We moved to work with NextStep in Redondo Beach, California (North of Newport) for an intermittent but impactful time. NextStep is run by Janne Kouri, who continues to be a strong force in the spinal cord injury community and who himself is an SCI survivor! Recently, he bravely wheeled himself across the country from the West Coast to the East Coast to raise awareness and funds for the SCI cause. Walking With Anthony refers SCI survivors to the many national locations of Janne's NextStep, which has been a remarkable resource to share. At one of our events, Walking With Anthony honored Janne for his tremendous contribution to the cause. NextStep provided Anthony locomotive training, which was important and functional in moving Anthony's legs. Locomotive training is critical in aiding the range of motion for anyone confined to a wheelchair.

In between these training sessions, Joe and I did extensive research searching for the best trainer available for Anthony's specific type of spinal cord injury. We found Mike Barwis of Barwis Methods. Mike is a strength and conditioning coach who specializes in spinal cord injury. We made a few trips to Plymouth, Michigan where the Barwis Methods is located so Anthony could work out directly with Mike. The journey from California to Michigan was taxing for Anthony but we knew the rehab relationship between Anthony and Mike was important. With Mike's assistance and a few of his own visits to California, Anthony had enough knowledge of the training he needed to do to continue his own workouts at home.

Every day at home, Anthony utilized what he learned and additionally leaned on the help of his cousin, Tommy, and especially his best friends, Bill Doody and Sean Swartz. Tommy put his life on hold and moved to California to be with Anthony at the beginning of this journey. The two are inseparable and have become close since the accident. Bill eventually moved in too, and Sean lived with us for an entire year to support Anthony and aid in his everyday workouts. The bonus of this loving support was a great motivation for Anthony. Mike continued to consult and coach Anthony with his training, guidance, and advice on rehabilitation equipment, which would liberate Anthony from requiring rehab at a third-party location.

Rehabilitation kept Anthony's body viable by building his strength and giving him goals to work toward. But we're still talking about a handsome young man of twenty-three who had been living life in the fast lane. He was driving a Mercedes, dancing at clubs, and basically having the time of his life and sitting on top of the world. Anthony had been living in Manhattan Beach, California with his friend Ben Greaves, also from South Florida, and both had been working for the Purcell family company business at Global Cash Card right up to the time of the accident. Here Anthony was, six months after our life changing moment, fighting every day to make great strides physically. Still, "tying your own shoes" wasn't much of a consolation prize for someone who exceeded in sports. His spirit was still very weak, he was depressed, and I was still very concerned. Don't get me wrong, through all this, his body was slowly gaining strength and gaining muscle memory back.

I now was fighting for the soul of my son's life—and that's why the idea of Walking With Anthony was so important to me. In hindsight, Walking With Anthony became the most important thing in Anthony's recovery as Project Walk eventually disappeared. I knew we had to aggregate more resources to help people in similar situations as my son. Despite the initial reservations of friends and family, my niece Tonya and I got busy with the very complicated and excessive process of paperwork that is required to establish a nonprofit. I had to use my own money initially to get the charity up and running, which I never hesitated doing. My attitude was pay it forward to others as a token of gratitude for all the strength and support Anthony and I received along this journey. In addition to money, Anthony, Tonya, and I devoted many, and I mean many, countless hours to the cause with the primary purpose of helping other spinal cord injury victims.

Setting up a 501(c)(3) is different from setting up a business. Setting up the nonprofit was a tornado of paperwork. Who's on the board? Are there conflicts of interest? State tax forms. Federal tax forms. Registries. On and on it goes. Thank goodness I had Tonya by my side— she really stepped right up to the plate to get this nonprofit moving forward. As I was always at Anthony's side, Tonya has never left my side during this journey. It's a tedious setup and sometimes it felt like we'd never finish just filling out all the forms and compliance statements. On the other hand, I've been an entrepreneur and businesswoman since I was sixteen, and I

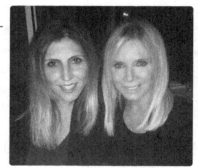

Tonya and Micki

do learn quickly and march forward with fortitude and an attitude into the unknown. Nothing was going to stop us, not even paperwork.

Coinciding with our time and involvement with Project Walk, they held an annual live-streamed event with a red carpet showcasing newly walking SCI survivors. Anthony and I were able to have a taste of these red carpets. My time in learning about all the families and their heartbreaking stories really paid off when they came to me to emcee their event. It was great practice for me when we began to venture into our own events.

When I saw the Project Walk red carpet full of the SCI victims in various stages of recovery, who spent the year working out at

Project Walk next to, and with, Anthony was a moment that really hit me. It solidified my belief that SCI victims can become healthier, stronger, and more independent through proper and swift rehab. Change needed to happen, and it needed to happen fast.

My friends who asked what I could possibly know about running a nonprofit soon learned the answer was "plenty." In just six months since beginning the tedious process, December 2010, Walking With Anthony was open for service. We were able to move the progress of the nonprofit faster than Anthony's own physical progress; however, once Anthony sunk his teeth into the nonprofit, his spirit renewed and la vita è bella. He began to see what a difference he could make for others, and it gave him a fire inside to keep up his energy for his continual physical workouts.

We learned that Anthony would need his full strength for what was to come. We held three major fundraising events over the next two years, which helped build up the funds we needed to accomplish what we set out to do — help and support other victims. Our first official big event took place in October 2011. I had the privilege of being one of the speakers at the podium, always thinking of Anthony to help keep my focus. We were chosen by the OpenField Foundation, a charitable organization led by former Green Bay Packers tight end Neil Wilkinson, to be one of the main beneficiaries of one of their Legends Fight Night events in Chicago. Their mission is to help organizations and individuals "striving to overcome tragedy, loss and/or grave hardship," which certainly describes Walking With Anthony to a tee. OpenField works with smaller, lesser-known charities like ours — organizations that by definition are underfunded or starting — to help us raise money through grants, individual donations, and help us raise our public profile. Tom Thibodeau, then the Chicago Bulls' head coach, was the emcee. This was just a few months after he was named the NBA Coach of the Year, so the turnout and enthusiasm was tremendous. Nearly 1,000 people came out to support our cause and Walking With Anthony was granted $50,000.

Anthony and I were blown away by the kindness, love, and support. Our whole family flew in from all over the country for this event, which made it even more special for Anthony. Walking With Anthony had just gotten off the ground, and we were already making a big impact and being recognized. Anthony could now see that he was more than his wheelchair and had a bigger purpose.

Being chosen by OpenField as a beneficiary really helped the launch of Walking With Anthony. Our grant allowed us to provide direct assistance to our first beneficiary, which was Project Walk. We wanted to pay it forward by donating them $10,000. It was the least we could do to pay it forward for their work with Anthony. We were honored when they named a new training room after Walking With Anthony.

The more I got involved with the SCI community, the more they got involved with us. When I think about it, that's how I discovered my calling. It was no longer just about Anthony, my son. It was about all of us—caregivers; brothers and sisters; moms, dads, and family; community; friendships, and above all, *real support when you needed it the most.*

The first official event planned, funded, and executed by our charity, Walking With Anthony, was called The Movement to Change. It took place less than a year after starting Walking With Anthony, in Los Angeles, at Siren Studios on April 13, 2012. Coincidentally, it was also my birthday. We quickly started this huge undertaking of booking the venue, reaching out to talent, and coordinating the theme. I was all in for making an impact, and this time Anthony was by my side and became my support.

It was a huge undertaking, but this wasn't going to be just another event—this would be a true Hollywood red carpet gala. Everyone was dressed to the nines. We're talking tuxedos and cocktail dresses. We were honored by the presence of a very close family friend, Jerry West, who most people know as the head coach and later, General Manager for the LA Lakers and today is a consultant for the LA Clippers, and his wife who is my dear friend, Karen. As they knew what happened to our family, (remember we were going to their Northern Trust Golf Tournament before turning back to

LAX the day of Anthony's accident), and they also wanted to support Anthony's cause. They had known about the accident since day one and had always been updated on Anthony's progress, so Karen soon became a board member for Walking With Anthony.

Also in attendance at The Movement to Change was legendary

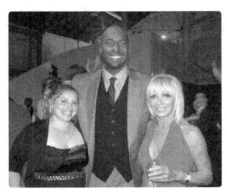

NBA veteran John Salley, who was the gala's emcee. John Salley had actually met Anthony several years prior at his daughter's birthday party—he later said that he was impressed by the fact that my son just sat down next to him and started joking around—so it was an easy ask to enlist John's support. In one interview with *Look to the Stars* (a website that shows which celebrities support what

Micki with Gigi Betancourt and John Salley

charities), John shared how impressed he was with Anthony's "perseverance, strength, and character." John went above the call of duty for Walking With Anthony and our first gala. He didn't just host our event, he spread the word around to anybody who would listen.

Jerry West and John Salley both spoke to the audience about the importance of supporting the work that our foundation was doing for SCI victims. I am still so grateful—in awe, really—of how everyone opened their hearts to us. I was living by my motto, "Bite off more than you can chew, and chew like hell." It took a lot of moxie to pull off an event of this scale for our foundation's first event! I put my money where my mouth was, and it was more successful than I could have ever imagined. The stakes were high because the suffering is insurmountable for victims, as is the cost of the recovery.

When your heart and head are in the right place, God shines through. I know an angel must have been watching over my shoulder that night, and Anthony's as well, because we wound up raising more than $100,000 for our mission. Even though Anthony was still healing and confined to a wheelchair, he was proud of the work he had just done for others. His soul was healing. Anthony began to slowly see a new future for himself and began making peace with God.

"I think anytime you call attention to a cause like this, it's an incredible thing," Jerry said to reporters on the red carpet during the event. "The cause is very special, and obviously Micki has done an incredible job of making a difference. She's taken it upon herself whereas a lot of people won't do things like that."

Jerry spoke eloquently about how important it was to bring SCI out of the darkness and raise public awareness of the struggles survivors and their families have to face. What I held dearly from that evening was the public acknowledgment of my vision and my efforts as such a compliment to have been supported. You never know the outcome of anything until you get there through your continual steps forward.

Not long afterward, in November 2012, we held the second Movement to Change event in Fort Lauderdale. This time, the theme was Time to Soar, which was a good fit for the venue, Hangar 9 at the Ft. Lauderdale Executive Airport. I enlisted family members, of course, and we all repainted the old airplane hangar with the Walking With Anthony's signature colors of red (courage and determination) and white (hope, spirituality, and possibility), and converted the whole place into nothing less than a nightclub. Speaker after speaker, including several SCI survivors, shared their stories of how they'd been helped by our organization. We honored the surgeon who saved Anthony's life, Dr. Allan Levi, Chief of Neurospine Service, at Jackson Memorial Hospital in Miami. Although his hospital time was a blur, Anthony never forgot the man who saved his life. It gave Anthony purpose to make this special acknowledgment at our event.

Spinal cord injuries can happen to anyone. It doesn't matter if you have money or not, if you are male or female, young or old, strong or weak. Former Buffalo Bills tight end, Kevin Everett, signed on as an honorary event chair. Everett's football career, as you may know, ended with a spinal cord injury—yet he refused to give up, and he has now recovered his ability to walk. I understood and connected with his perseverance. His story was so impactful that everyone in the room was crying as he shared his story of struggles, successes, and life changes. I watched Anthony out of the corner of my eye as he heard the story too. Anthony gained more determination that day and carried his head a little higher than he had for the past two years.

The Time to Soar event was an even greater success than the original Movement to Change gala, raising more than $150,000 for our foundation. This was also the first time Walking With Anthony officially began awarding grants and handing out awards as part of the formal ceremony. Our foundation was thrilled to give Nick Williams and Chris Hickox, two graduates of Anthony's high school who also had spinal cord injuries, grants of $10,000 each to attend Project Walk. Anthony was able to reach out to these two who shared similar backgrounds with him. It connected him to the life he once knew with the new life he was now living.

Since then, we've given out $10,000 grants at every event. It's incredibly moving. These are people facing dire circumstances, and that grant not only provides financial relief, but it's also a reminder that they are valued, that they are loved and that they are important. Everyone needs a little light in their life, but with the frequent isolation of spinal cord injury victims' experiences, it's even more important. It's also a lot of fun for Anthony because it's always a big surprise; the heroes we help don't know they're receiving the grant. I do contact the recipient's parents to let them know, but other than that, we keep it really *hush-hush*. I wish I could share with you their faces when Anthony, in his wheelchair, hands them a check. They are surprised and go totally crazy. They connect with him instantly. Truly, this is Anthony's favorite moment of his charity involvement.

The success of the Movement to Change fundraisers led me to thinking we could still do more to change lives. Ideas started to form in me, and I was inspired to do a golf tournament. Why golf? Not only do I play golf, but I already had a great venue in mind—the Country Club of Fairfax, Virginia, a family Country Club that my sister Frannie and my brother-in-law Bernie McKeever are members of. Every time I am in town, I take over the course with my large personality. I knew that Anthony was ready to take on a bigger challenge as well.

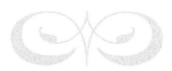

2 Corinthians 4:8

"We are afflicted in every way, but not crushed, perplexed but not driven to despair, persecuted but not forsaken, struck down, but not destroyed."

CHAPTER SEVEN

Expanding Our Reach

All systems are go with the Nolan family running Walking With Anthony, especially my niece Tonya, who is the administrator and, of course, Anthony and I. When we have the opportunity to put on our events, the entire family rallies around me to help. Even with the early success Walking With Anthony had, we still didn't have all the resources to help everyone who needed it and meet the demands that the SCI community needed. We would receive (still do) forty plus calls, letters, or applications a month. It's like a tidal wave that Tonya, Anthony and I would work tirelessly to address regularly. It's at least $100,000 a year for a single month of rehab for one person. That's just to get them out of the chair and learning to get healthier, stronger, and more independent. That's a monumental achievement in and of itself for the victims. And we know, spinal cord injury victims simply cannot do it alone—it's nearly impossible for most people. The calls for help come into us for all different types of needs but always with the same sense of urgency.

One hectic moment I vividly remember is when my sister Terry and I were running errands and dealing with all of the last-minute planning for our early Siren Studios event—making sure the entertainment was sorted and produced, that catering received their final deposit, and we reviewed the final menu. Even the arrangement and rearrangement of the guest list and seating placement is something that is dynamic up until the moment the doors open. I wasn't even close to being dressed for the event.

In the middle of all this, I received a distraught phone call from a mother, Crystal Dixon. I slammed on the brakes of the event to turn our attention away and attend to her needs. This is what we do now — we attend to the crisis at hand. We were six hours away from the start of the red carpet arrivals for our gala event, but this mom needed to be heard.

"Calm down, calm down," I requested of her.

The irony of me soothing her to calm down when we were finalizing last-minute details and trying to get ourselves dressed and ready to receive our guests wasn't lost on me.

"Tell me what's going on." I invited her to continue.

Crystal was crying into the phone as she shared with me her son's story. This was the first time I ever heard it, so I gave her all my focus. At only thirteen years old, Donnovan was left quadriplegic from a spinal cord injury when he was tackled head first at a Pop Warner youth football game in Long Beach, CA. He'd been a star player who had just moved up to the league's Junior All American level.

Crystal worked in a grocery store, one of the lower-wage jobs that gave little to no benefits. All of her co-workers donated to Crystal their personal vacation and sick time so she could take the time off to take care of her son. But eventually, she had to go back to work because she needed to maintain her son's health insurance for his care.

She didn't have any family nearby. She was completely alone taking care of her son, the whole nine yards—you know this repetitive story. She had reached the point where she couldn't pay her rent or buy groceries because all of her money went to keeping her son alive.

"Crystal, who do you bank with?" I asked.

As she gave me her information, you could practically hear the tires shrieking as I brought the fundraiser planning to a dead stop, and did a sharp U-turn to the situation at hand. Seriously, what does putting on a gala event do to help SCI victims if we can't be present enough in the moment to help one of our own—right then, right now!

Terry and I jumped in my car and went directly to my bank. I didn't want to take any chances with an electronic transfer, she needed the money now. I made my withdrawal, got back in the car and drove directly to her bank for a cash deposit that covered her rent, her groceries and a little more. Some might say this was out of character for me—we all know how driven in the moment I can be when I'm planning or working on a project—but as the mom of someone with SCI, I know that sometimes there are things that just can't wait or be put on hold. What was a few minutes at the bank when someone's life was at stake?

Donnovan's story was particularly sad because it shows just how badly families can suffer, especially when there are children involved. Crystal ended up suing Pop Warner due to the mechanics of the game he was being taught when the injury happened. But in the meantime, this didn't help them live day in and day out with his condition.

After a couple years, Crystal had to go back to work in order to keep what insurance coverage she had for Donnovan and the lawsuit continued. With no one to turn Donnovan's body regularly, he got bedsores, which eventually required what was supposed to be a routine surgery. This surgery took place just months after they finally came to a legal settlement and were working toward better-ing their situation.

At eighteen years old, Donnovan died unnecessarily on the operating table of complications from a surgery that could have been prevented if there had been help available for Crystal and Donnovan. No amount of money can replace her child, but Crystal has honored his memory with a foundation of her own, Donnovan's Dream. Additionally, what happened to Donnovan helped add better practices to Pop Warner, which, even though can no longer help him, will hopefully prevent more injuries like his to other children.

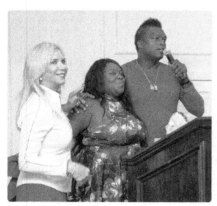

Micki, Crystal, and LaVar Arrington

It's experiences like Crystal's that keep the fire in me lit, that give me the nerve and strength to approach big personalities like those that work within the Washington Redskins organization. As we know, this is something that affects so many of their players, year after year.

The Country Club of Fairfax is one of the most prestigious clubs in the Washington, D.C. area. Frannie, her husband Bernie, and I, were always treated like royalty by the incredible and generous staff. We decided Walking With Anthony would become an annual event in September. This was the month we needed to raise awareness as it made the most sense. Not only is the weather perfect and people are ready for a weekend getaway, but September also happens to be Spinal Cord Injury Awareness Month. I just needed a partner to help make this new venture a reality and the biggest impact to create change possible.

I did a ton of research and found Tommy Fitzgerald of Nesconset, New York, who's been associated with JetBlue's Annual

Author's NOTE: *Throughout this book, you will read about how Walking With Anthony has partnered with the Washington Redskins organization. At the time of this printing, the team has temporarily changed its name to Washington Football Team; however, due to the timeline of when the book was written, the organization is still referred to as the Washington Redskins throughout.*

Swing for Good Golf Classic charity tournaments for years. Tommy was exactly the person I was praying for. His mother was diagnosed with multiple sclerosis when he was still just a boy, which really sensitized him to the struggles physically disabled people face. Later, when Tommy was an adult, a co-worker's child was diagnosed with leukemia, and this propelled Tommy to organize his first charity golf event to help defray their medical costs. Those costs had to have been astronomical for the family. Tommy's been holding these events ever since and has literally raised millions of dollars through thousands of these golf tournaments for a variety of charities.

After many reach outs, my persistence paid off. I was able to connect with Tommy on the phone to share our Walking With Anthony story, our mission, our struggles, and our successes. Most importantly, I was able to emphasize how far Anthony had progressed in his rehabilitation, and how we learned through his experience that rehabilitation was the best passageway for spinal cord recovery. Tommy was thrilled to learn of the grant recipients that benefited from Walking With Anthony, which highlighted an interest for him. He understood the value of the charities work and the need to help more SCI victims. We ended up talking for a long time, pitching ideas and concepts, and finally, he agreed to participate with us for our tournament. He's been with us ever since. I'm extremely humbled to have him be a part of our team.

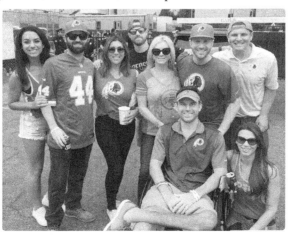

During a planning lunch meeting, the conversation came up about how the Nolan and Purcell families were huge Redskins fans.

"Look, we've got to go get the Redskins to be our partner," he declared with excitement.

Quizzically, I responded, "What do you have in mind?"

A team in the making, with my *won't take no for an answer* attitude and Tommy's passion for this commitment, we were eventually able to get a meeting after much back and forth and a little convincing. Our fifteen-minute allotted meeting with Jerry Olsen, the Executive Director of the Redskins Alumni Association, turned into a ninety minute meeting in the Executive Conference room full of passion, ideas, and support. In all my hopes for Walking With Anthony, I never imagined this materialization of partnership.

Before I even knew the meeting was over, Jerry stood up and announced, "I'm all in and we'll bring in the alumni association for support. This is exactly the kind of cause we want to be involved in as a team," and he also noted, "Spinal cord injury is a real threat to all NFL players."

As Tommy and I vacated the building, I could barely feel my feet touch the ground. I genuinely felt like I was floating on air. It was such a validation of my vision, coming from none other than Jerry Olsen that what I was trying to do for SCI victims was significant and was greater than just Anthony and me.

This news would ignite Anthony's recovery beyond imagination. I couldn't wait to share the news with him. Like the rest of our family, Anthony is a big Redskins fan. When he found out that he was going to be meeting with former players, he immersed himself even deeper into the work of our non-profit. Yes, it would be fun for him, but he knew that they would bring more attention to something that was truly important to him. He was ready to make change for others.

Anthony hit cloud nine when he learned that Terri Lamb, President of the Washington Redskins Cheerleaders Alumni Association, also signed up in support. That grin on Anthony's face lasted for weeks. She's honestly been a godsend, supplying every one of our golf tournaments with all of the help and volunteers we could ever need. The First Ladies of Football Cheerleaders help out with the event, handling everything from registration to handing out gifts and acknowledgements on the field. My family, whose been stretched putting on these mega events ourselves, has now found their dream team with all the additional support we could imagine. Our team was building, and our mission was spreading.

Jane Rodgers was our next advocate to join and support Walking With Anthony. Jane, at the time of our meeting was the Executive Director of the Redskins Charitable Foundation. She has led many wonderful initiatives such as providing washers and dryers to low-income schools and community centers throughout D.C., so impoverished children could have clean clothes for school. She worked through the Redskins Charitable Foundation to provide sports equipment to inner-city schools and empower young women and girls to reach for and achieve their dreams. Jane really helped get me off and running by practically holding my hand while introducing me to everyone. Today, we're like family.

Saying that Anthony was excited about the involvement of the Washington Redskins Alumni and the Washington Redskins Charitable Foundations in our humble charitable organization is an understatement. He was beaming with pride for weeks as we worked alongside these high impact figures. In fact, it still brings a smile to his face, and he looks forward all year to our event. It keeps his spirit going even through his dark times.

Every year, I attend the Redskins' official events where I have the opportunity to stand up and speak about Walking With Anthony. I meet all the players and schmooze 'em. It's my opportunity to share what I've learned through my experiences with Anthony and how far along he's come. A dinner event at team owner Dan Snyder's house, while speaking about Walking With Anthony, resulted in an invitation to sit on the leadership council of the team's Redskins Charitable Foundation, which I gratefully accepted.

The team's presence made our first tournament absolutely monumental, and every event since continues to mean so much more to Anthony, my family, myself, and Walking With Anthony. Since its beginning, our golf tournament has only gotten larger, and has made more impact each year. Anthony works hard to share his story and the mission of our charity to anyone who listens. Each event brings more and more Redskins players to the tournament than

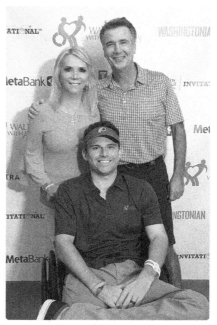

Micki and Anthony with Bruce Allen, GM of the Washington Redskins

the previous. We've even had Bruce Allen, the former team president of the Washington Redskins attend. The team's sideline announcer Rick "Doc" Walker — a former NFL player turned radio sports commentator — is our annual event emcee. As a former pro football player himself, he understands the importance of rehabilitation for SCI victims so he hosts his local ESPN radio show live from our charity golf tournament. Larry Michael, the former "Voice of the Washington Redskins" has even blessed us with his presence. He invites me to be on his local NBC sports show every year.

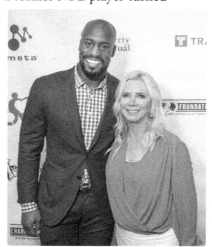

Micki with Vernon Davis

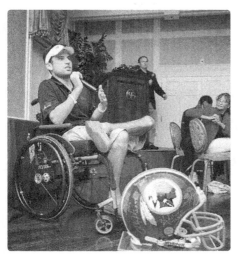

We've been able to form a true Washington Redskins partnership especially with playes such as LaVar Arrington, Jeff Bostic, Mark Mosley, Vernon Davis, Mike Bradd, Roy Jefferson, Charlie Taylor, Mike Nelms, Darol Green, Doug Williams, Alfred Morris, and Pat Fischer. Many former athletes have seen their careers end prematurely after a spinal cord accident. It is truly heartbreaking, and so it stands to reason, that team owners and coaches, as well as other players, want to give back. They have seen the pain and struggle firsthand. We could not be more blessed with everyone's participation.

Despite Anthony's injury, Anthony has said that going through this struggle has made him a better person. Kinder. Stronger. More empathetic. More tolerant and patient. I see it every day in his interactions. He's the first to lend a hand, an ear, or a shoulder to cry on. He may have had a terrible accident, but his spirit grew stronger, and his sense of purpose was renewed. I am proud of the man he has become.

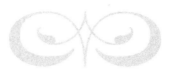

Romans 8:28

"We know that in everything God works for good with those who love him, who are called according to his purpose."

CHAPTER EIGHT

Lasting Impact

Today, Anthony is Mr. Walking With Anthony, the executive director of our charity. My son, who had once been suicidal, now shares his story often and persuades other victims out of their own suicidal thoughts. He's grown to become a mentor to other SCI victims, showing them that there is a future after paralysis

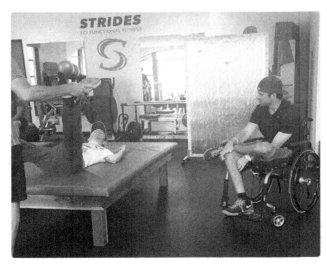

Anthony mentoring another SCI victim during physical fitness.

and they have more to live for even if they can't live the life they once did or thought they would. Anthony doesn't walk, but he is still a walking miracle—and he's become a better person since the accident, of his own admission. It's about getting healthier mentally in addition to physically. Stay healthy, stay strong, and remain independent. Be of service. Live a rich and meaningful life of purpose.

Many people thought I was crazy thinking I could start a charity, including Anthony. I'm just fierce and determined to find the *good way* of a situation. Since establishing Walking With Anthony, we've given out close to $3 million dollars to cover the costs of rehabilitation for both short- and long-term caregiving. We don't keep a dime. Not one person at Walking With Anthony draws a salary of any kind.

I've worked with other organizations, and it usually takes something like twenty people to get an event off the ground. When you see the quality of our events, you would never have guessed that we started with just a handful of family and close friends, all done *pro bono*, free. Each and every one of us has put our heart and soul and faith into form from the very beginning, and it's amazing to witness its growth. The money we raise goes directly to SCI victims who need it right away. We provide a community of love and support, where people facing enormous odds and unimaginable struggles can find others who've shared a similar experience, who can offer advice, counsel, or just listen. We lift up and celebrate every success story, and we mourn everyone who stumbles or falls along the way.

If there is one thing I have learned through this journey with Anthony, it's that no one can do anything alone. They say it takes a village to raise a child—well, it takes a much bigger village to help someone who's suffered a spinal cord injury. Nearly one in fifty people have a spinal cord injury that has left them with limited or no mobility; that is nearly a half million people. Another 10,000 people are similarly injured *every year*.[6]

---

6 https://www.christopherreeve.org/living-with-paralysis/stats-about-paralysis

Of special urgency was the Disability Integration Act (DIA), introduced to the Senate early 2019, which per the Congressional Bill: "prohibits government entities and insurance providers from denying community-based services to individuals with disabilities that require long-term service or support that would enable such individuals to live in the community and lead an independent life".

When victims are forced into institutions they often lose all their freedom. As one of the litigants who won the right of integration said, the DIA "enshrines in Federal statute the right to live in community. It gives people with disabilities and seniors the right to demand that states and insurers remove the obstacles which stand in the way of their own integration." It's nowhere near to becoming a law at this time.

However, it is essential that the Americans with Disabilities Act (ADA) remains in force. Passed into law in 1990, the ADA protects individuals with disabilities and helps them live as full-fledged members of society. We all can thank the ADA for wheelchair access at public and private places, for the handrails in bathroom stalls or for the curb cuts that allow people with limited mobility to do something as simple as crossing the street without help from someone else. It also ensures that they aren't passed over for a job and are treated the same as you and me, and are provided with the accommodations they need to live ordinary lives, and are seamlessly integrated into society like everyone else.

We need these laws to ensure people like Anthony, and all our heroes in the next chapter, can live full, rich lives as valuable and valued members of society. If you don't have a family member who's dealing with a spinal cord injury, it's very difficult to imagine these barriers. We take for granted the fact that we have handicapped spaces for parking or in restrooms. Yet even with these laws, so many places don't even have access to the so-called accessible bathroom! I can't even begin to count the number of restaurants where I went out with Anthony and wound up saying "they don't have a ramp, not wheelchair accessible, guess we can't go in today."

Some states offer financial assistance through the Catastrophic Illness in Children Relief Fund (CICRF). In New Jersey, for instance, their CICRF is a state financial assistance program for families whose children have an illness or condition otherwise uncovered by insurance, State or Federal programs, or other sources, such as getting help from fundraising. Imagine being in a state that doesn't offer this, knowing you need it and that you would qualify for it. I imagine it's heartbreaking.

You would think that handicap discrimination wouldn't be an issue anymore or that places would ensure easy and complete access for those in wheelchairs. But I see it all the time, and if you start looking, you will too. When an issue shows up in front of me, my family and I have to take a stand. This is a great way to make a direct impact that anyone can do and helps to ensure that another survivor can thrive in everyday life.

To the point, my family and I were visiting my mother who had a trip and fall accident at her apartment in Ocean City, Maryland, and this was a glaring issue. All the Nolan wagons circled to support mom, and especially Anthony, who was really excited to see his grandmother. Upon arrival, we then realized that the elevator was not handicap accessible. We had no way to get Anthony to the elevator. We were only surrounded by stairs everywhere. This is a community of senior citizens, people in their seventies and up! Outrageous! With Anthony, I knew we had to advocate for the senior citizens.

I have to admit here, I was a maniac that day. I got upset in front of Anthony in the parking lot. It flustered me that not only was my son unable to go upstairs to visit his grandmother, but after all these years of fighting for this cause my own mother's building wasn't handicapped accessible by lift. The residents were coming out of their doors and peeking out from behind the curtains as they heard my screams of unhappiness. They must have thought a crazy person was on the loose.

"Are you kidding me?" I remember ranting. "This place needs to be wheelchair accessible. What is wrong with the management of this place? It's a senior citizen's community for goodness sakes."

"That's just not right," I vented.

Anthony was embarrassed as he already felt burdened by the predicament, but I was unhappy. We'd come all that way, and my mother was excited about seeing him. For this entire trip, Anthony was left out from seeing his grandma. As a society, we still haven't caught up to the expanded needs of our disabled.

There are so many codes and regulations to protect the independence of disabled people—things that we don't even question or bat an eye at—that it's shocking when you see some places trying to get away with doing the bare minimum, or perhaps less.

We had a similar experience at one of our favorite restaurants in the same city of Ocean City, Maryland. When we visit annually for our July 4th Nolan Reunion, we go to this little place called The Crab Bag, the best crab shack in the city. We'd been going there for years and never thought about the handicap accessibility at the restaurant. Now, after Anthony's accident, it suddenly became a whole new reality for us. In order for Anthony to get into the restaurant, he had to use this rickety, shaky lift. It was scary as heck just to look at the thing, never mind trusting it to lift an adult man in a wheelchair. It was honestly just plain dangerous.

Stop for a second and consider how vulnerable our modern world is from the perspective of living in a wheelchair. It makes us stop and hold our breath to consider what someone else is going through when they may not have the right means to do something like go into a restaurant safely. It became too much for me to continue allowing Anthony going up this shaky lift. It was just unfair for him to go through. As his advocate and his champion, I finally had to complain to The Crab Bag.

"This is crazy!" I exclaimed to the manager. "This thing isn't safe in any way, shape, or form. Why hasn't it ever been fixed? You know my son comes in here by way of wheelchair."

Sometimes I say a lot and I say it loud. But it's like physically disabled people don't even exist to people with full mobility and someone has to be their voice. It's a blind spot to able bodied people. You just don't see it until you go through it.

I'm happy to share that the owners listened, understood, and responded. Gold star for The Crab Bag! When we visited the following summer, they had installed a beautiful, very wide, cement ramp. Anthony and I love to continue eating there. Anthony never feels out of place as getting in and out is seamless and now second nature to him. There is no staring as we don't struggle to get him in to enjoy our favorite Chesapeake Bay crabs.

These stories hopefully shed a little light on why the ADA is important for people like Anthony and anyone else with limited mobility. There's an entire section of the act, Title III, which deals specifically with public accommodations for the disabled. It covers everything from hotels, restaurants, stores, schools, hospitals and even doctors' offices, golf courses and stadiums. One would think that a doctor's office or hospitals would make accommodations already, but I've learned through the years that nothing will get done without laws in place.

The ADA also specifically provides tax credits and write-offs for businesses making those improvements. There is no reason any business should not follow what the ADA lays out to ensure a productive and independent life for a disabled person. However, we see issues, such as how often enforcement of the laws are loose and businesses get away with not worrying about a large population that they don't see. Even digging to see worse, we can see where it can be parasitic when troll attorneys fine businesses for the slightest thing out of line. I'm talking an inch off of specified dimensions. I simply ask that we stop and think about the world from the physically limited perspective as we share and manage space together. Let's ensure that we do things correctly the first time and make changes when appropriate.

I am continuously looking for a single chain store that directly advocates and is consistent in their accessibility for the disabled. Other than the specified building codes, franchises on a whole don't go out of their way to ensure comfort for the disabled. It's even worse when it comes to the airlines. Airlines are not even comfortable for able-bodied people, imagine how it is for someone in a wheelchair. The government is aware of the airline issue, which almost makes this issue worse.

There's a specific law for airlines to ease the burden for flying for people with disabilities, the Air Carrier Access Act, and from my experience, at least with Anthony and the people Walking With Anthony has worked with, it's rarely enforced. It is supposed to protect disabled people from any discrimination when flying and also to accommodate their needs in a professional, timely, and most of all, respectful manner. But what we see are people strapped into the front of the plane like cargo, long waits for access to wheelchairs, often damaged equipment, and don't even think of going to the bathroom like everyone else in a timely or reasonable manner. Of course, I get this is a delicate situation; it's an airplane, and it's already a tight squeeze. There is no excuse for bad policy that doesn't even come close to the spirit of the law, never mind just treating disabled people with a little more dignity.

It's bad enough when ordinary people are ignorant. They typically can be taught. They can learn. But politicians in D.C. just seem to make it worse. As recently as 2018, Congress attempted to pass legislation that would have gutted the accommodation provisions of the Americans with Disabilities Act in the guise of "reforms." These so-called "fixes" would have forced people with disabilities to jump through a whole bunch of new hoops before getting their day in court. At the same time, the bill would have changed the requirement from "providing access" to making "substantial progress" in providing access. Why would our politicians change the fact that businesses need to require access? The people behind this laughable "reform" bill were a bunch of lobbyists operating on behalf of corporate realtors, who put saving a few dollars ahead of compassion for people in wheelchairs or who are otherwise limited in their mobility. This would have been a major step backward, and thank goodness the bill died in the Senate.

A lot of people don't know this, but one of the saddest ironies of spinal cord injuries is that politics treat it like, well, a football - thrown around a lot. Take stem cells, still one of the most promising paths to a permanent cure for spinal cord injuries that I've researched and learned about. In 2001, then-President George W. Bush placed tight restrictions on federal funding for human embryonic stem cell research, which is a very polarizing topic in the public. He was widely criticized by many spinal cord injury advocates, including the Christopher Reeve Foundation, for what's seen as bowing to political lobbying. His successor, then-President Barack Obama, overturned those restrictions. The Supreme Court declined to hear a challenge to the new policy, but recent changes made by President Donald Trump about fetal tissue research are calling those gains into question again.

We see it time and time again, lobbying and money in Washington, D.C. deciding what happens for people with disabilities like choosing a hot or cold drink of the day. Rarely—if ever—do they hear the voice of actual, real people. In the end, for many issues and laws that are put into practice, I just don't care what party is sitting in the White House. I do want our elected officials to see what life is really like to instill real changes and ensure those changes are made and made quickly for the benefit of SCI victims.

In the meantime, there is still work being done on all other levels in a variety of ways, such as the Christopher Reeve Foundation's Big Idea Project. From what I've seen, this trial shows some real promise— although it's still in the experimental stage—using implanted epidural stimulators to help SCI survivors move their limbs, bear weight, regain bladder and bowel control, and even sexual function.

We've also worked with NextStep, which is working to open paralysis recovery centers across the country to ensure that people with SCI can access physical therapy, research-based interventions, and reliable care. Walking With Anthony has referred many of our of SCI victims to various NextStep facilities around the country.

It's a full court press at every level to ensure SCI victims get the help they need because accidents aren't going away.

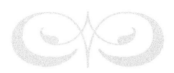

Hebrews 4:16

"Let us then with confidence draw near to the throne of grace, that we may receive mercy and find grace to help in time of need."

CHAPTER NINE

Our Heroes

What is a hero? As Anthony and I discuss throughout the year our upcoming event, we take to heart the process of selecting our upcoming SCI hero where Anthony will have the privilege of honoring our hero on stage at our annual tournament or gala. Our heroes come from many different backgrounds, but each has exemplified courage as they all survived their personal injury and are working toward a thriving future.

The following heroes have all been honored at our past events:

Name: Rachelle Friedman

Hometown: Virginia Beach, Virginia

Favorite Hobbies: Playing with her daughter, blogging

Date of Injury: May 23, 2010

Level of Injury: C6 spinal cord injury

Our organization's first hero was Rachelle Friedman, who you may have recognized at one point in the news, as her personal story gained national attention. Rachelle was at her bachelorette party horsing around with her friends. Goofing around, an unidentified friend playfully pushed Rachelle into the pool just weeks before her dream wedding, where she hit her head on the bottom and was instantly paralyzed from the neck down. This is the story every parent has sleepless nights over, worrying that this could happen to their child.

Rachelle suffered a C6 spinal cord injury and was told those fated words by her doctor, "You will never walk again." Clearly, that doctor didn't know Rachelle's personality, candor, or strength. Very quickly, though, she ran out of her insurance's outpatient rehabilitation like most with spinal cord injury, and was not receiving the necessary rehabilitation required. The medical neglect had Rachelle falling under 100 pounds. She became extremely weak with low blood pressure.

When Anthony and I first learned about Rachelle, I immediately reached out to her and her family. She was desperate for rehabilitation services, so Walking With Anthony flew her out from her home in Virginia Beach for ten days to go to Project Walk where she received the help she needed. At that time, Project Walk and Walking With Anthony were still partner organizations. We also covered her transportation and her housing expenses through

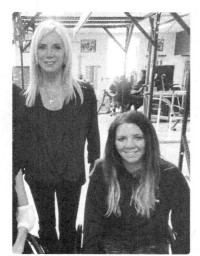

Walking With Anthony, which ended up costing about $10,000 for a week.

Rachelle has been a celebrated Walking With Anthony hero since 2012. She married her betrothed Chris Chapman and the two of them haven't looked back. She went on to write about her own accident in her memoir, *Promise: A Tragic Accident, A Paralyzed Bride, and the Power of Love, Loyalty, and Friendship,* which became a Lifetime Television movie.

Rachelle's gone on to be one of the most visible and strongest faces for SCI survivors, with tens of thousands of followers on social media and a TLC Documentary about her inspirational journey. She's gone on to be a writer and mommy blogger, a motivational speaker, a mom, a reality show star, even a surfer.

Through everything that she experienced, Rachelle still dreamt of having a picture with her newborn daughter where she would be standing. With the support of her family, through her training, stretching and workouts she was able to do just that. Her daughter Kaylee is now four and a half years old, and Rachelle and Kaylee are inseparable. Rachelle is almost completely independent and is now considering if she and her husband should add another baby to their family!

Rachelle and Chris will be renewing their vows on their ten year anniversary, as well as her ten year *quadiversary*. Her final dream would be a redo bachelorette party. I know it's going to happen, and it will be perfect for her. Anthony and I will be by her side in whatever support she may need as she has always been one of our strongest supporters. Not only does she come to all of our events, but she also helps make the events happen. Oftentimes, I'll find her working the phones to get sponsors. As she has received many blessings, Rachelle truly believes in giving back, and we are so grateful for her continued friendship.

Name: Nick Williams

Hometown: Fort Lauderdale, Florida

Favorite Hobby: Wheelchair Tennis

Date of Injury: May 4th, 2008

Level of Injury: T2/T3 spinal cord injurys

Nick Williams was a schoolmate of Anthony's; he was talented in volleyball and dreamed of leading his team to a state title. Nick and Anthony both went to Cardinal Gibbons High School in Fort Lauderdale, FL.

Early in the morning on May 4th, 2008, Nick was driving to pick up his uncle from his mom's condo in Fort Lauderdale to take him to the airport. Nick's uncle had been in town to watch Nick play in the district championship volleyball game. It had been one of the biggest games of his life.

However, during the short distance drive, Nick struck a tree and a street sign in the median of the Federal Highway going between 45 and 55 miles an hour. He was taken to N. Broward Medical Center where his family was informed he might not make it.

Instead, Nick survived and was in a coma for two weeks. Once he woke up, he found himself paralyzed with both brain and spinal cord injuries. He eventually moved to Jackson Memorial for their spinal cord rehab program where he lived for the next three months to start his new life.

He was told he'd "never walk again." Nick has since used leg braces to help him maneuver. He won't listen to the negativity that is sent his way by either doctors or anyone else. Anthony has continued his friendship with Nick, and they both understand the difficulty in bouncing back from an athletic life.

In 2012, Walking With Anthony presented Nick as a beneficiary with a $10,000 grant for Project Walk in Orlando for a month. His family encouraged and supported him to stay longer, so he ended

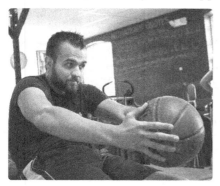

up staying there the rest of his summer. He made tremendous strides in his recovery during this time.

Doctors never thought he would be fully independent or be able to go back to school, but he proved them wrong. By working hard and never giving up, he graduated from college with a degree in communications and a minor in political science in 2017. Nick was hired right out of college working at a mortgage firm as well as a substitute teacher at his alma mater Cardinal Gibbons High School.

God also must have some very important matters for Nick Williams to take care of in this life as well. As luck or misfortune would have it, while in his wheelchair, Nick moved underneath a tree during a rainfall while reading a Bible verse from the Bible app on his cell, but then was struck by lightning, and his wheelchair caught on fire. Neighbors rushed out quickly, and the first responders were quick to the scene. Still, he died from a heart attack in the ambulance at twenty-eight years old, but was revived four minutes later by paramedics. Then Nick fell into his second coma for four days and woke up once again in a hospital.

He spent about two months in the ICU and when he was well enough, moved to the Neuro rehab to relearn how to move and use his body again. Luckily, his muscle memory had survived from all his hard work at Project Walk, and it gave him a good starting foundation. Burn marks have left an imprint of his wheelchair on his back and head, but he is alive and has a strong spirit burning in him.

In 2019, Nick was celebrated at our annual golf tournament that he was unable to attend, and so he watched Anthony's speech from his hospital bed. He recently left Ryder Trauma Center of Jackson Memorial Hospital with his loyal girlfriend, now fiancé, Emily Netter. He continues to go to physical therapy five days a week at three different places: Neurofit 360, Spectracare, and Ronni's Sports Medicine. He also does physical therapy through hyperbaric treatments to ensure he is living his best life. Go Nick, keep defying the odds and thrive!

Awesome first day of Project Walk!!! Hard work gets it done!! Thank you Micki Nolan Purcell, Anthony Purcell, and Walking With Anthony for this opportunity.

— Nick Williams

Name: Erica Predum

Hometown: Fort Wayne, Indiana

Favorite Hobbies: Anything with my kids/family and concerts/music shows

Date of Injury: May 14th, 2007

Level of Injury: C5/C6 spinal cord injury

Erica Perdum was driving home from work with her youngest child in the car when she hit the rumble strips on the side of the highway. Overcorrecting, she flipped her SUV, which rolled over several times, and was thrown from the car. Her son, thank God, was strapped in securely and didn't get hurt at all. Erica, however, suffered a severe spinal injury. She was airlifted by helicopter to the hospital, where she went through a series of emergency surgeries. That's when she found out that she was paralyzed. She suffered a C5/C6 injury, leaving her unable to move from the chest down. She has arm movement as far as her wrists are concerned, but Erica is confined to a wheelchair. She went through the typical thirty day rehabilitation and then the hospital simply sent her home to *figure things out*.

About eight years ago, Erica was on Facebook looking for crowdfunding therapy sessions at Project Walk, which as we know, is really expensive. That's when one of her friends in the spinal cord community mentioned Walking With Anthony, and told her to reach out. She had already been paralyzed for twelve years and had all but lost hope when I met her. Her mother had been her primary caregiver. When Erica's mother died of brain cancer, Erica was left in an even more difficult predicament, alone with her two young boys to care for.

When Anthony and I heard her story, we knew we had to help. One of the first things we did for Erica was gifting a handicapped accessible truck to her so that she could care for her two young children.

Meanwhile, my personal worst fear became Erica's true nightmare. Erica's doctor was prescribing her pain medication that she ultimately became addicted to. According to the National Institute of Drug Abuse, 8-12% of opioid prescribe patients will misuse their medication for their chronic pain. Erica said she had no idea how addicted she had become, but her doctor continued to give her more and more of the medication. At one point, she actually overdosed which almost took her life. More than 130 people die every day from opioid overdose.[7] Erica was in rehab for almost a year kicking the drugs. In fact, her addiction cost her her kids as she was declared an unfit mother, making the spinal cord injury secondary to the need to clear the addiction.

Erica suffered loss after loss after loss after her car accident. She called me in desperation, frantic and upset, especially over losing her right to mother her boys. I called her attorney right away. Walking With Anthony covered her legal bills to represent herself and her recovery to the courts as a fit mother. Thank goodness, following her recovery, she was successful in getting her children back through the proper legal means afforded to her.

Overprescribed pain medication is an absolute crisis in this country. After Erica's fight for her sobriety, she eventually won on both fronts. She won her freedom from the dependency of the pain meds and she won her sons back. Today she doesn't need or use any medicine for pain management and has found her own alternative health options such as meditation and prayer. Meanwhile, as her sons have grown older, they've adapted well to life with their mom in a wheelchair and with their mother's paralysis. When her home health aides aren't there, the boys help tuck her into bed, help her into and out of her wheelchair, and all the tasks you'd expect living with a spinal cord injury family member. She admitted to me that when things get frustrating—and we all have those days—she reminds herself and the boys that they are all a team and this is what their family looks like, one hand washes the other.

---

7 https://www.drugabuse.gov/drugs-abuse/opioids/opioid-overdose-crisis

Erica has found normalcy as a single paralyzed mother raising two boys. She credits her community and her church in Texas for really surrounding her and her boys with assistance, affection, and attention, making life easier. She says she has so much to live for and like me, we believe in family and faith.

She is a strong woman. She'll be the first to tell you that having a spinal cord injury is pure hell—but she's also the first to say that if you keep pushing through the challenges, it does get better. Walking With Anthony, Erica says, has become like her family. She also regularly and freely checks in with me or Anthony whenever she has a hard time. Devoted to Walking with Anthony, she recently drove eighteen hours with her brother, Randall, and her best friend, Cas-

sandra, to our most recent charity event in support of our cause. She hasn't missed one event we have ever had. I'm the one who gets to be humbled by these sheer acts of courage and commitment. Now, she is in her second year of college! Erica is a true hero!

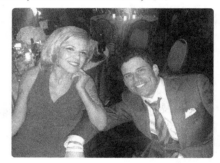

Name: Marccello Castillo

Hometown: Springfield, Virginia

Favorite Hobbies: Xbox, Video Games, listening to music, going to concerts, hanging out with friends

Date of Injury: October 15th, 2018

Level of Injury: Acute Myelopathy with Chronic Spinal Cord Stenosis

Some of the hardest times for Walking With Anthony are when we receive stories about children. It's a terrible burden for any parent,

I can personally attest, but it's harder when your child is underage and still has much to experience. They also don't typically fully understand their situation and their mentality is more fragile than an adults on why something is happening to them in this extreme. Any parent would rather switch places with their child to end their child's suffering, as watching a child suffer physically, mentally, and emotionally is heartbreaking. Anthony and I do everything we can to offer support in finding the best care and technological advances to help these children, which is the least we can offer back to a community that has also done so much for us. Marcello Castillo, and his mother Guissela, are part of our family now.

In 2019, our honoree for the Walking With Anthony Charity Celebrity Golf Tournament and Dinner was one tough kid, a fourteen-year-old named Marccello Alvarez. At our 7th Annual Charity Celebrity event with our 300 attendees, our handsome young Marccello was the recipient of our financial grant that went towards a brand-new wheelchair accessible van from our partner, Mobility Works, along with Jim O'Meara who worked tirelessly to make this happen. We proudly raised over $200,000 that evening.

Marccello has had spinal problems since day one as there were unfortunate complications during his birth. He had his first spinal decompression before he was even two years old, and the doctors told Guissela that her son would never have a normal life. They informed her that Marccello would never be able to walk or talk, and predicted that he'd spend his life in a vegetative state. Marccello—who was eventually diagnosed with a rare genetic condition called chondrodysplasia punctata, which is a skeletal disorder that affects his arms, legs, and spine—wound up proving the doctors wrong. Though he was always weak, he was no vegetable. He was smart and while he had limited movement, he could take care of himself.

He had gone through another spinal decompression at around five years old and surgery terrified him. By the time Marccello made it to school age a year later, he started developing some muscle weakness, which became alarming. It turned out that due to a combination of continual neglect and mistreatment at school, Marccello sustained an injury by a school caregiver. His C1 and C2 vertebrae started to curve, forcing his neck to turn backward—and as a result, his brain was collapsing. Marccello would need surgery. However, being the intuitive mother that she is, Guissela could tell that Marccello simply wasn't mentally or emotionally ready for surgery just yet; instead, they went to the National Rehabilitation Center (NRHC) for intensive therapy. Years later, as Marcello turned fourteen, is when Guissela and I connected.

Guissela told me that by this point they were praying that their insurance would at least cover Marccello's wheelchair. They needed bathroom renovations because Marccello couldn't even move anymore. They also needed a van because he was too big for Guissela to put in her car by herself. Detail after detail shared by this mother described a life that was being forced to do a full 360° change.

"I understand completely," I said. "The most important thing right now is you need to keep your son happy. You have to keep Marccello motivated, you need to keep his spirits up, so he'll keep fighting. That's the most important thing, Guissela."

"What does Marccello like to do," I asked. "Does he have a pastime or a hobby?"

It's important for children with a spinal cord injury to have an activity, no matter how basic, to keep their minds—and to any extent possible, their bodies—occupied.

"He loves video games, but right now he can't really play," Guissela replied. "He can't move his hands or arms, and it has completely devastated him." She added that Marccello was depressed because he also couldn't talk on the phone or text his friends. He had become completely immobile; this wasn't the life he knew. She described to me how the rehab center staff let him use a headset that allowed him to play games and it also connected him with other people who were playing the games too. However, with a nearly $4,000 price tag for the device, this was simply out of her reach and believed by her to not be a necessity in the abundance and ongoing checklist of items needed to care for Marcello.

I disagreed. There's a freedom for a child like Marccello to escape into his video game world where he can experience what he can't experience in his physical body and connect with others on an equal playing field. Microsoft is one of the leaders in bridging the gap for people with limited mobility playing games through ground breaking technology. Many people saw this technology for the first time during the 2019 Superbowl for their Microsoft Xbox Adaptive Controller. This is life changing technology for children. It is single handedly one of the biggest things that can give them a sense of normality.

"Okay, you need that for Marccello, because it's very important," I insisted. "I'm going to get him that headset equipment, and anything else that he needs."

We made a plan with the young female therapist at Marccello's rehab, who was cool, hip and young enough to know exactly what

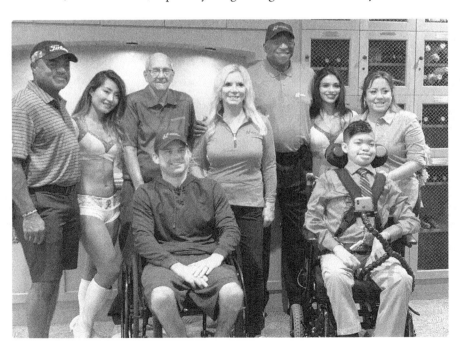

Marccello would need for his gaming. We wired her the money to order all the equipment and Marccelo got his game ON! His spirits turned positive instantly.

Their family already had enough to worry about, and this was an important investment of a few thousand dollars from Walking With Anthony. We were able to honor Marccello at our most recent event. Our event celebrated Marccello like the king he is, with TV cameras interviewing him on the red carpet. Guisella was over the moon, and Anthony was beaming. Anthony did the speech and awarded them with the much needed van. He was the best person to understand the battle Marcello had fought and connected with him instantly. It was a full house and a full standing ovation by everyone in the family. I was honored to help this family keep their faith that things could get better.

———◆———

Name: Daniel Mowery

Hometown: Boca Raton, Florida

Favorite Hobby: Going to the gym

Date of Injury: November 17th, 2018

Level of Injury: A C4 Complete injury

I love spending time with my daughter, Jennifer, and her family when I am in Fort Lauderdale. She keeps me busy from morning to night with my grandbabies. In 2018 while visiting, Jennifer shared with me details about a man who was rumored to be, "rotting in the hospital from an SCI injury."

The next day, Jennifer and I drove like gangbusters to Broward Health North. Turns out, Jennifer knew all too well.

In my determined way to get things done, I marched right past the nurse's station into the hospital room of a handsome young man, the same age as Anthony, named Daniel Mowery. His mom,

Michelle, a single mother, was sitting there holding his hand while he held on to his dear life. With very little support from the hospital, she was washing him, changing him, catheterizing him, and flipping him, every two hours. She was living at the hospital with him.

This mother willingly shared with me his story. On November 17th, 2018, Daniel Mowery had been heading toward a great life. He was starting a new managerial position and was heading out to the gym for his daily workout when he was in a bad motorcycle accident on Federal Highway. Daniel was hit head on by a car going the wrong way that caused a burst fracture to his C5 vertebrae pushing into his spinal cord with a diagnosis of a C4 complete injury.

The lack of skill at this hospital had resulted in Daniel losing over thirty pounds in just six weeks. The caseworker was always pushing back on Michelle when she attempted to have Daniel moved to a more appropriate facility. She didn't have the energy or the stamina to keep pushing back as his advocate.

When I got involved, it took some time for the hospital to release Daniel's medical records to his mother. Once his mother was finally granted access, I immediately sent them to my go-to doctor, Dr. Allan Levi, right away. He said that Daniel's surgery was performed correctly but that now we needed to get him into rehab right away.

I arranged an ambulance to come free of charge and to waive their high fee for a next day transport of Daniel to Brooks Medical Center in Jacksonville, Florida for a three-month stay at no cost. Daniel is making outstanding progress, and we were happy to have Daniel featured as one of our upcoming honorees as he certainly is one of our heroes. His bounce back to life when he went into rehab was life changing. Anthony understood the difficulty of transitioning from a state of not moving to grueling physical rehab, but he knew it was worth it in the end.

We are grateful that Walking With Anthony can be a positive influence in someone's life, such as Daniel's, following a tragic accident. We were very happy to provide him one of the best spinal cord

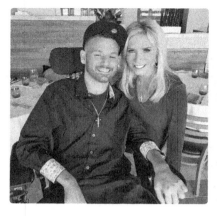

injury rehabilitation options, and continually offer moral support in any way we can. He now continues to work out in Miami. He is working hard to get a grant to continue at Grant Medical, which we are always here to ensure he does get.

Walking With Anthony has been a positive influence in my life since my accident. They were able to help get me accepted to the best spinal cord injury rehabilitation I could ever imagine, Brooks Medical Center in Jacksonville, FL. They have been by my side since they were informed about my injury and have been a positive influence and offer great moral support. I owe a lot to them & I am thankful for them every day.

— Daniel J. Mowry Jr.

Name: Chris Norton

Hometown: Altoona, Iowa

Favorite Hobbies: Speaking, Running his own Non-Profit, Raising his Family

Date of Injury: October 16th, 2010

Level of Injury: Fractured C3, C4

Chris Norton, the 7th Annual Walking With Anthony Golf Tournament honoree, is an inspiring and motivating former football player. Anthony and Chris have many things in common, including the type of injury and the year of their injury. He spoke eloquently to the attendees about his personal battle defeating the odds after suffering SCI during a college football game.

During the third-quarter play in a football game against Central

College in Decorah, Iowa on October 16th, 2010, Chris's head collided with the ball carrier's knee during a kick-off return. The impact fractured Chris' C3 and C4 vertebrae on the spot. As you often see in football games, the pile cleared and Norton laid motionless on the ground face down. Without a peep from the crowd, he was transported off the field by ambulance and taken to the emergency care facility of Winneshiek Medical Center where doctors stabilized him enough to be able to airlift him to the neighboring Mayo Clinic.

Oftentimes, I am asked why we partner with football. My answer is always: there are a lot of SCI injuries in football. When Chris

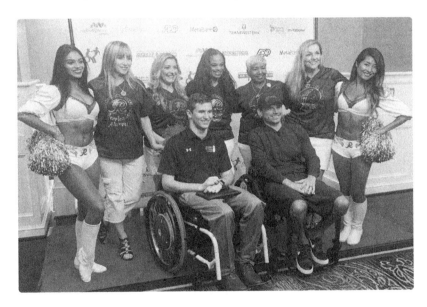

was paralyzed with the same injury as Anthony, he had a 3% chance of survival or the possibility of living with no movement or feeling from the neck down. Like Anthony, Chris, had the means to fight to get better — money and advocates. He regained mobility throughout his body including his hands, legs, feet, and torso. He also recovered significant sensation in his lower body.

Chris's progress has been so significant that he was determined, and then able, to walk across the Luthor College stage on May 24th, 2015 with the help of his fiancée, Emily Summers, to accept his diploma in Business Management. The inspirational and motivating video went viral, notching over three hundred million views.

Then, during the spring of 2018, Chris and Emily, who met each other online, married in Jupiter, Florida, exchanging vows from his wheelchair after he walked slowly down the aisle, seven yards to be exact, with Emily's support. The ceremony was filmed by *People* Magazine. Chris and Emily went on to write the book, *The Seven Longest Yards: Our Story of Pushing the Limits While Leaning on Each Other*. There has also been a documentary made about them, *7 Yards*. Be sure to keep your eyes open to watch their inspirational journey.

Chris and Emily have gone on to adopt five girls and have fostered over seventeen children. Today, Chris is a well-known motivational speaker. From his home in Florida with his family, he runs his own non-profit foundation, the Chris Norton Foundation, and they are continually doing amazing things for the SCI community!

———

Anthony and I have witnessed so many success stories and have been following other SCI victims and their progress that we celebrate when we receive texts, phone calls, emails like the following:

> *Walking With Anthony provided me an awesome opportunity to participate in the Cyberdyne Hybrid Assisted Limb Rehabilitation Program in Jacksonville, Florida. I was unsure if I would have been able to participate in this program until WWA was able to provide the financial assistance I needed to do so. Since this program, I feel a much stronger neurological connection between my muscles and nervous system & better form while walking. Walking With Anthony helped me take the next step on my journey to walk again, and I am forever grateful.*

— Sean Mahoney

However, this work never stops.

On the other side of the spectrum, I received the following text from a family member, and realized our work continues:

> *Hi Aunt Micki! I have a friend Amanda who is a pediatric resident at Broward General and she has a 16-year-old patient who is paralyzed (quad) due to a disease called transverse myelitis and she reached out to me to get more info about WWA. Can I pass on your email so she can get some more information to see if maybe WWA would be able to help? Which email should I give her? Thanks so much!*

———◆———

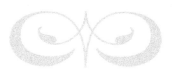

James 1:12

"Blessed is the man who endures trial, for when he has stood the test he will receive the crown of life which God promised to those who love him."

CHAPTER TEN

In the End, There is Only Love

My granddaughter Makayla was very little when Anthony became paralyzed, and my two other grandchildren, Mackenzie and Matthew, weren't even born when Anthony's life changed. They don't know Anthony, their uncle, outside of his wheelchair. They only adore their uncle, shower him with love and kindness, and they only see Anthony as Anthony is - which is

Uncle Anthony. They don't see him with pity or regret. Anthony has multiple wheelchairs in his home, and when his nieces and nephew are visiting, they all get into the wheelchairs and wheel around with him. For me, it's pretty cute to watch. This is the

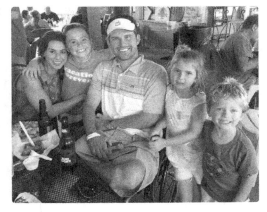

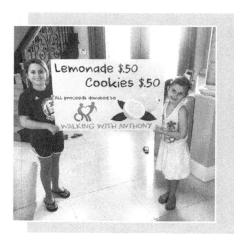

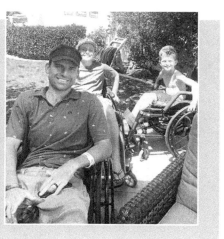

same innocent lens that we should all view handicapped people with.

My grandchildren even took it upon themselves to raise money for Walking With Anthony. They had a lemonade stand in their neighborhood and raised $100, but of course, being my grandchildren, they took it even bigger. My grandkids attend Saint Coleman's Catholic School at Pompano Beach, Florida, the same grade school that Anthony had attended. They created a fundraiser in which the students contributed a dollar to Walking With Anthony. Once contributed, they would be excused from having to wear their uniform to school the next day. I don't know if my grandchildren get their business sense from me, or if it's a family thing, but those kids have a real interest in raising money to help others. They ended up raising $10,000.

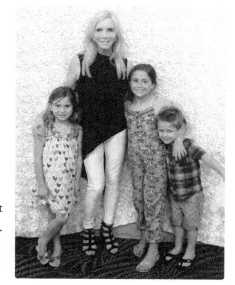

Anthony was doing well for himself working for our Global Cash Card business before his accident; he was a very integral part and was one of the best salespeople. Today, he enthusiastically oversees our new financial services company, Roundtable Financial Group (RT Financial), as our Chief Operating Officer. Anthony has always had a sharp mind in business and is thriving within the company. He has bounced back to much of his former self. Just like with the charity, Anthony 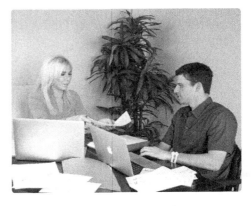 completely immerses himself day in and day out into his work. A wheelchair has not stopped his life from moving forward. He's working the phones, closing deals, and running the whole show. Anthony had been groomed by his father to run the company where he can showcase his natural-born leadership skills. RT Financial is Anthony's business and Walking With Anthony is his passion.

Even though Anthony doesn't walk today, Anthony is my walking miracle. He continues to become healthier and stronger every day. When he started his physical therapy, he didn't have any upper body strength. I mean none at all. He was as weak as a baby; no wonder, he'd been paralyzed from the neck down and his muscles had atrophied. Today, he has his whole upper body strength back. He works out constantly with free weights, barbells and dumbbells, working on his pectorals, delts, lats, and biceps.

He eats incredibly healthy: protein, fruits and vegetables. He won't touch soda and only drinks water. He avoids carbs at all costs. Anthony is very strict about taking vitamins. His one vice, if you want to call it that, is a nice cold Bud Light on the weekends. He won't touch it during the work week, but come Friday evenings and Saturdays, there's nothing he likes better than having a beer with his buddies and watching football on the big screen. Overall, Anthony has turned into a total health nut, and I'm grateful for his strict mentality that keeps him focused. It's really easy to lose all your muscle tone when you have no mobility so you don't want to eat something that is a detriment to your body as you already have a daily uphill battle to fight.

Anthony lives out our Walking With Anthony mission every single day. One of the most powerful things I witness him do on a continual basis is mentor others struggling with spinal cord injuries, paralysis, and limited mobility. He shares his personal story, his struggles and how hard he's had to work to regain his life back. He's always been excellent in front of an audience — I've often told him he should be a motivational speaker, and now, in a strange way, he is, but on a more personal level. He gives people hope when they need it most. He's a lifeline to children and adults in despair. He is sometimes their light in the dark. If there's one thing we've learned from dealing with Anthony's injury it is that it's not just about staying alive: it's about living your best life, and living it as best as you can, no matter your circumstances.

And love walks in…

Karen Unis was one of Anthony's high school classmates at Cardinal Gibbons, Fort Lauderdale, Florida. My understanding is they weren't particularly close in high school—just casual friends who shared a couple of classes together —but, I believe she always had a crush on him. Whenever I mention this to her she always laughs at me. She reached out to him on Facebook once Anthony was in California starting our new life after the accident. Ironically, Karen moved out to California right after college where she pursued a career as a dental hygienist around the same time. They began talking on the phone on a daily basis, as Karen kept checking in on Anthony, offering him words of encouragement and continual kindness. It was exactly what he needed, and you could see the change and impact she was making in his life as his confidence kept building.

There was one challenge Anthony was having trouble facing; he was still embarrassed about being in a wheelchair, and for the longest time he refused to meet her in person. He was still trying to come to terms with what had happened to him, and didn't feel like he was the person he used to be, nor the person she once knew. He hedged and delayed, hiding in his own insecurities. This was a time that he was still emotionally fighting the battle of what happened to him and shedding the life he once knew. Still, Anthony's resistance to going beyond their daily phone calls eventually became a deal breaker for Karen.

She gave him an ultimatum, "If you don't meet me in the next two weeks, I am done."

I can still understand why Anthony was shy—his life had been turned upside down—but it seems to me like Karen gave him the kick in the pants he needed. He finally agreed to see her in person.

The day came for the two to meet in person. Anthony picked out a casual but chic outfit, put on the cologne that hadn't been used in a year, and gave himself the cleanest shave. I could see that Anthony was a nervous wreck while he anticipated the evening to come. He was so nervous about seeing her again that I noticed he didn't eat the entire day. Remember, this is the man who had contemplated suicide, but was now fighting butterflies in his stomach. I already knew he was in love as I watched him be stir crazy at home all day. For moral support, Anthony was decked out with his full entourage in tow, which included Jennifer and Matt along with my nephews Tommy and Kyle, and nieces Tonya and Kellie, who all tagged along on this first date. They chose the very eclectic Roger Room in Los Angeles to have a drink.

Being a nosy mom, Frannie and I were around the corner at another hotel—no one wants their mom for a chaperone, especially when you're an adult. Still, Tommy was texting us every detail of what was going on.

Tommy: Getting cozy talking about a homecoming game.

Tommy: She just ordered a Mai Tai and moved closer to him.

Micki: 💜💜💜

Tommy: THEY JUST WENT OUTSIDE TO THE PATIO TOGETHER.

Most importantly, we heard the romantic details on how Anthony and Karen looked at each other throughout the night. It was clear to me, even through these texts, that these two had a real connection.

Tommy texted me that the two had gone out on the patio to be alone, at the Four Season's hotel. *They're kissing now, they're kissing now*, read the texts. I was literally jumping up and down at the hotel doing the happy dance, we were so excited, and cheering at the top of our lungs. If anyone had seen us, they would have thought I won the lottery. To me I did. I was so happy for my son to have this huge chance at love in his life.

Karen and Anthony married in October 2017 at the Pelican Resort in Newport Beach. As we always do, we went all out to throw the biggest event possible. Every single family member and friend was in attendance. This was the happiest day of his life, and mine and Joe's. From that day, they haven't been apart since. Karen always says she never sees the wheelchair. They support each other through ups and downs. A love story made in heaven. Anthony may have not lived the life he expected, but the life he is receiving has exceeded his expectation. Love does heal. God doesn't always give us what we want, but God gives us what's right for us.

With this union, I hope to share more grand-baby photos with you. Thank you so much for journeying with me through Walking With Anthony.

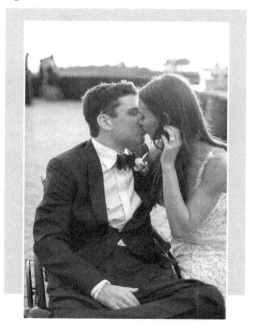

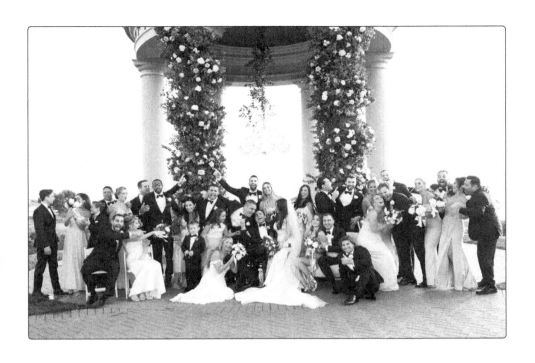

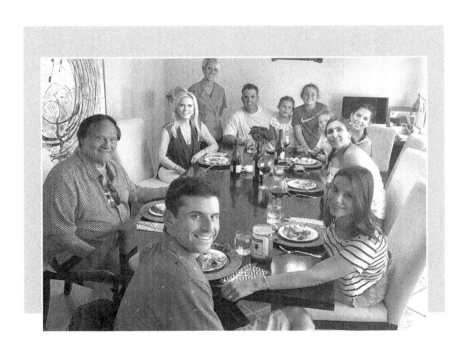

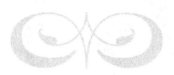

John 10:14

*"I am the good shepherd. I know my own and
my own know me."*

EPILOGUE

I was born in Washington, D.C., the third of eleven children: Pat, Terry, me, Joanne, Frannie, Bernie, Chrissy, Tommy, Barbara, Billy, and Katy. Soon after, our family moved to Bowie, Maryland, a middle-class suburb located just east of the nation's capital and about fifteen minutes west of Annapolis. It's one of the three largest cities in Maryland today, but when I was growing up, it was just a tiny little place.

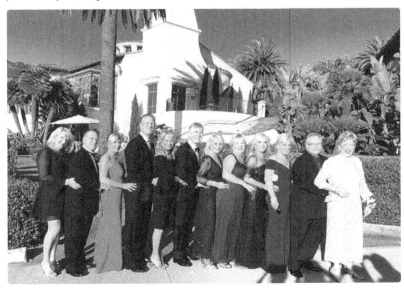

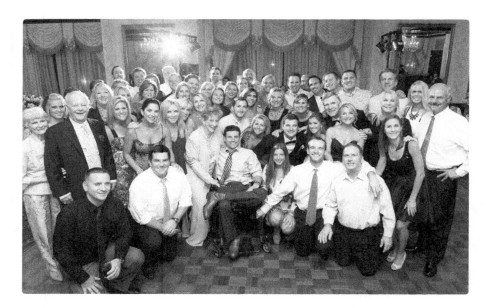

I don't know what it is like to be from anything else but a large family. Each of my brothers and sisters is unique in their personalities, but I have always had the largest personality within the family, an outgoing, adventurous, "I can take on the world" approach to life.

My siblings and I are close in faith and family. To this day, my brother Bernie texts all of us a daily spiritual meditation every morning. We are all on one text thread. We pray for each other. We celebrate each other. We even comment on the mundane aspects of each other's lives. If anyone has a problem, we all pitch in. My oldest brother has a heart condition so we all pitched in to install a lift in his home to help him with the stairs and to ease his burden.

Two of my sisters struggled with alcoholism and addiction. We worked really hard as a family as we rallied around them to get sober. In fact, we pulled both my sisters back from their addictions. As anyone knows, getting a family member sober is not an easy task. We are genuinely one of those families that sticks together through thick and thin, through good times and in bad. Fighting for a family member is nothing new for me—and you'd better believe memories of fighting for my sisters helped drive my fight for Anthony. I wasn't shy to push someone to be their best or to push them when they couldn't push themselves.

My father, on his deathbed, made me promise never to sell the dream house that we bought for him in Ocean City, Maryland next door to his brother. We bought this house for him in 1977 to keep the family traditions going as we have two family reunions a year that absolutely every family member comes to. Dad started the 4th of July celebration, and my sister Terry, also in Maryland, hosts the Thanksgiving gathering under a tent in her backyard that sixty-plus family members joyfully attend.

My mother has made the biggest impact on my life. She has inspired me both as a mother and a business woman. I have witnessed her own success and growth as a person. Not only has she impacted me, but I see her impact on our entire family. Even this year, when my mother couldn't make the 4th of July dinner celebration because she had an accident, we made sure to include her through Facetime. Every single grandchild would have a chance to speak with *Gigi*. My brother, Pat, always gets things going with the family congratulations. He celebrates who has graduated or other special events that a family member had that year.

On Thanksgiving, we each write something we're thankful for on a small piece of paper and mix them up in a bowl. All the little grandchildren read it, and then we all jump in and try to guess who was thankful for what. You might laugh, but listen, this keeps all the little ones from getting in trouble because there are too many of us paying too close attention.

Terry was always the rock growing up. She's the one you could depend on 100%. She took on our mother's role. She would have long intellectual conversations with my father. Terry also made sure everyone would do the household chores. When my mother went to work, she would write on a large poster board everyone's chores. To this day, Terry still complains about the responsibility she had on her when she was young, but it's safe to say she is an amazing sister and a wonderful woman.

If Terry was the reliable one, I was the wild child. As a teen-ager, I was the one who snuck out at night to have adventures, running all over the place. For some, it's hard to stand out in a crowd—as a teen, I longed for my own independence, and it was no surprise that I left home almost as soon as I graduated. I was only sixteen years old when I moved in with a friend from high school into our first apartment. Those were fun times with a lot of great memories. I remember we had this yellow shag carpet and a big white leather couch.

From a very young age, I was exposed to a lot of things. I worked hard. I played hard. I traveled all over the place. It was my first time living on my own as an adult, spreading my wings and feeling my oats — I had an absolute blast. I also started my first real job. I was off and running—my family only saw me for Sunday dinner, which was a ritual we all enjoyed and I never missed. Family has always been my anchor, and still is today.

I never had the desire to go to college, and I didn't have the money to go anyway. However, my high school had a special program for senior year students, in which I got to work for a local company. Such a wonderful opportunity for an ambitious kid like me. It allowed me to get school credit while building up the employment experience I'd need to support myself as an adult. What I learned has lasted a lifetime.

I signed up with Bel Air Engineering in Bowie, Maryland, and by the time I graduated, I had a full-time job with the company. My boss saw my potential and took me under his wing. Soon I was learning business principles: how to read a P&L sheet, budgeting, management skills, how to talk to people, and everything else you'd need to know to run a successful enterprise.

Moving on to bigger things, I headed for Washington, D.C., looking for work in the city. It is an enormous and confusing metropolis, the kind of place where you're just one more face in the crowd—but I wasn't. I was sitting in yet another waiting room at yet another employment agency, Washington International Secretarial Exchange (W.I.S.E.). Many had told me there was no work available, but I persisted. I could hear the owner and his staff talking to other job applicants on the phone and thought to myself, *I can do this, I know I can.* Finding jobs for people to do? That was easy. I knew how to manage people from my days at Bel Air Engineering.

I walked right up to the owner and asked for a job on the spot.

"I don't have any openings," he began, but I cut him off.

"Look, I'll work for free," I said before he could shut me up and show me the door. This was probably the last thing he wanted to deal with, some hard-driving young woman like me who wouldn't take no for an answer.

"You don't even have to pay me anything until something comes up," I continued. "All I want to do is sit and listen to you, to learn as much as I possibly can."

Taken aback by me, and unsure of where I was coming from, he responded hesitantly,

"Okay, if that's what you want to do, let's try it,"

What did he have to lose? It's not like I was going to cost him anything. I was already working nights as a waitress. I'd work through the late night hours, and then show up at the employment agency every morning and began learning everything I could. I have a crazy work ethic—everything I do, I give 150%—and I was soaking up information like a sponge. I had the energy, and the time, and I didn't want to waste either. I was stimulated and enthused by all that was happening. About two weeks after I started, one of his employees left to do missionary work in Africa. Suddenly, I found myself with her desk, but more importantly, her Rolodex.

I'm a hard charger: I leveraged that Rolodex and all its contacts to the hilt, and I soon became the top job recruiter for the agency. Eventually, I wound up running the entire company before being made Vice President. I was driving a new white Cadillac at the age of twenty and then I started my own business when I was twenty-six. Communication and connecting people is a strong feature of myself that I don't take for granted.

Working for that employment agency was what ultimately brought me to a staffing industry convention in Chicago, where I met my husband Joe Purcell, Anthony and Jennifer's Father. He swept me off my feet. Within six months we were married, and I moved to Los Angeles where he lived. He was king of the staffing industry in LA with several offices.

Joe told me I didn't have to work, but I had other plans.

"I want to open up an employment agency," I told him. I knew that I was good at it, and I enjoyed it.

Beverly Hills was home to my new office. Soon I was in business as M.N.P. Personnel (Micki Nolan Purcell Personnel) with just the Yellow Pages and myself. I convinced my sister Frannie to come out and work with me.

I built up MNP Personnel to become one of the largest employment agencies for high-level executive assistants. I still run into people today that I placed into job positions years ago. Even just recently, I had dinner with a woman that I placed in a job in 1984.

After many years of marriage, Joe and I divorced, but our working relationship continues to thrive. One of our most successful ventures together, outside of our children, was our launch of Global Cash Card. Joe and our children, including Joe's sons from his previous marriage, Joseph and Michael, built Global Cash Card together into one of the largest payment card companies in the world. Our solution gave the unbanked a debit card with the ability to have payroll deposited to the card. There were so many benefits to using our card that the employees and employers both loved it. We started Global Cash Card in 2003 and Global Cash Card was sold in 2017 to ADP.

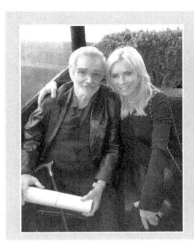
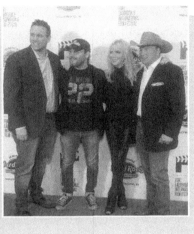

In addition to being Executive Vice President of our new family business, Round Table Financial, I also get involved in films as an Executive Producer. I've always loved the Entertainment Industry. It was really exciting to be involved in Burt Reynolds final film before he passed away, The Last Movie Star.

Many of my ventures end up becoming successful because of all the energy and hard work I put in, whether it's a business enterprise, philanthropy, film production, or investing. I relied on that exact same spirit, diligence, and philosophy that I've had my entire life

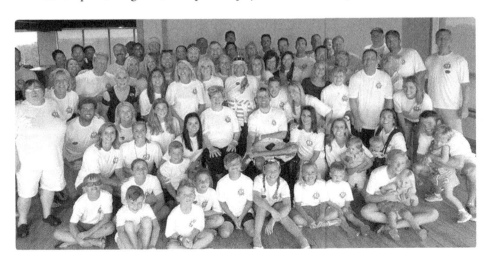

when I turned to establish Walking With Anthony. I'm not saying it was easy. And I'm not saying we didn't have our struggles. Whenever I'd get frustrated, or angry, or feel like I wanted to give up, I'd think of Anthony and other spinal cord injury victims, and I continued to push forward, as they are my inspiration. The struggles of the SCI are so much greater than anything I have ever dealt with—it is their fight, their aspirations, their hopes and dreams that keep me going, that still keeps me going every day.

I encourage everyone to find a way to reach out to someone with spinal cord injury. More often than not, they may feel alone and want someone to connect to. If you are able, please donate time or money to an organization, such as Walking With Anthony, to help SCI victims get the help they need to survive and thrive. I'm glad I was there for my son.

www.WalkingWithAnthony.org

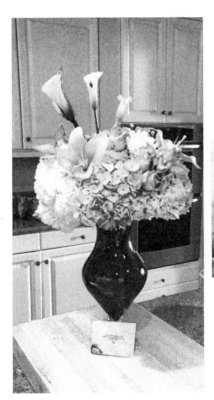

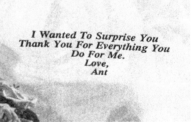

*I Wanted To Surprise You
Thank You For Everything You
Do For Me.
Love,
Ant*

A true story of triumph over tragedy. At this time in history, it's one thing to rise to occasion for her family but another to recognize the needs of others. Micki is a prime example of acting in the best interest of community over self. A beautiful and inspiring story.

Janne Kouri
President and Founder
Next Step Fitness

Paralysis is an affliction that displaces the life of its victim and decimates the family that surrounds them. Micki Purcell has lived through the atrocities faced by a parent when their child's life is changed forever. A seemly hopeless circumstance that she met head on with an unwillingness to submit to its consequences. In doing so she has not only impacted the life of her child but the lives of many who face the atrocities of the system that leaves them helpless. Through this book, she illustrates there is always a light in the world if we are willing to see it.

Mike Barwis
CEO Barwis Corporations
Director of Sports Science Detriot Red Wings
Senior Advisor Sports Science New York Mets

Walking with Anthony is a spot-on representation of a determined, loving mother's holistic approach to helping her son Anthony overcome his physical, mental, and spiritual struggles. A mother's love so strong, it helped her son push through his struggles with suffering a spinal cord injury and now continues to overflow into the lives of other families who are living through similar SCI struggles. My personal spinal cord injury experience was dealt a very similar hand as Micki described Anthony's, and I desperately needed additional support. I encourage anyone to read Walking With Anthony to gain insight and an accurate perspective of what a mother's love can achieve when faced with her child's life-changing tragedy.

Erica Predum
Walking With Anthony Hero, C5/C6 Spinal Cord Injury

Micki Purcell is a whirlwind of positivity and her Won't Take No For An Answer Attitude is part of the formula for success which she models for any family to overcome SCI. This heart-wrenching and heart-warming story will educate you and inspire you to advocate and get involved with helping families with SCI loved ones.

Louise Phipps Senft
Mother of Archer, SCI c2-c5 burst ASIA A Complete injury 2015

Published by

TVGUESTPERT PUBLISHING

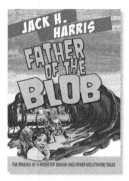

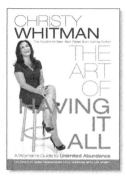

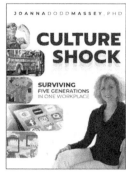

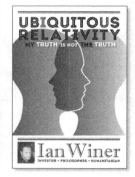

JACK H. HARRIS
Father of the Blob:
The Making of a Monster
Smash and Other
Hollywood Tales
Paperback: $16.95
Kindle/Nook: $9.99

New York Times Best Seller
CHRISTY WHITMAN
The Art of Having It
All: A Woman's Guide to
Unlimited Abundance
Paperback: $16.95
Kindle/Nook: $9.99
Audible Book: $13.00

JOANNA DODD
MASSEY
Culture Shock: Surviving
Five Generations in One
Workplace
Paperback: $16.95
Kindle/Nook: $9.99

IAN WINER
Ubiquitous Relativity: My
Truth is Not the Truth
Paperback: $16.95
Kindle: $9.99

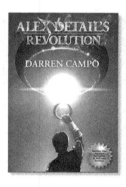

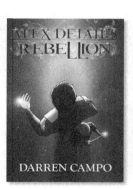

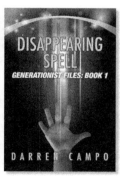

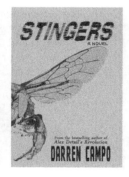

DARREN CAMPO
Alex Detail's Revolution
Paperback: $9.95
Hardcover: $22.95
Kindle: $9.15

DARREN CAMPO
Alex Detail's Rebellion
Hardcover: $22.95
Kindle: $9.99

DARREN CAMPO
Disappearing Spell:
Generationist Files:
Book 1
Kindle: $2.99

DARREN CAMPO
Stingers
Paperback: $9.99
Kindle: $9.99

TVGuestpert Publishing
11664 National Blvd, #345
Los Angeles, CA. 90064
310-584-1504
www.TVGPublishing.com

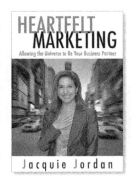

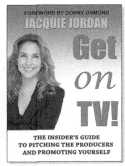

JACQUIE JORDAN AND
SHANNON O'DOWD
*The Ultimate On-
Camera Guidebook:
Hosts*Experts*Influencers*
Paperback: $16.95
Kindle: $9.99

JACQUIE JORDAN
*Heartfelt Marketing:
Allowing the Universe to Be
Your Business Partner*
Paperback: $15.95
Kindle: $9.99
Audible: $9.95

JACQUIE JORDAN
*Get on TV! The Insider's
Guide to Pitching the
Producers and Promoting
Yourself*
Published by Sourcebooks
Paperback: $14.95
Kindle: $9.99
Nook: $14.95

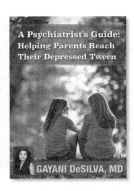

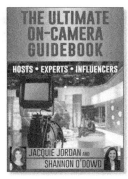

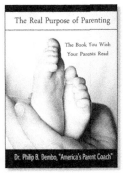

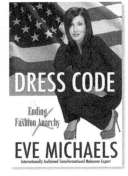

GAYANI DESILVA, MD
*A Psychiatrist's Guide: Helping
Parents Reach Their Depressed
Tween*
Paperback: $16.95
Kindle: $9.99

GAYANI DESILVA, MD
*A Psychiatrist's Guide: Stop
Teen Addiction Before It Starts*
Paperback: $16.95
Kindle: $9.99
Audible: $14.95

DR. PHILIP DEMBO
*The Real Purpose of
Parenting: The Book You Wish
Your Parents Read*
Paperback: $15.95
Kindle: $9.99
Audible: $23.95

EVE MICHAELS
*Dress Code: Ending
Fashion Anarchy*
Paperback: $15.95
Kindle/Nook: $9.99
Audible Book: $17.95

- spine source of support
- Insurance, $, who pays for SCI